Asthma

Management in Primary Care

Robert Pearson

MSc MB ChB MRCP D.ObstRCOG

General Practitioner, Stratford-upon-Avon
Clinical Assistant in Chest Medicine, South Warwickshire Hospital
Medical Tutor, Asthma Society Training Centre, Stratford-upon-Avon

RADCLIFFE MEDICAL PRESS
OXFORD

15 Kings Meadow, Ferry Hinksey Road, Oxford OX2 0DP

British Library Cataloguing in Publication Data

Pearson, Robert
Asthma: management in primary care
1. Man. Bronchi. Asthma.
I. Title
616.23806

ISBN 1 870905 45 8 (hardback)
ISBN 1 870905 40 7 (softback)

Printed and bound by Billings, Worcester
Typeset by Advance Typesetting Ltd, Oxfordshire

Contents

	Acknowledgements	*v*
	Foreword by Donald Lane	*vii*
	Preface	*ix*
1	Anatomy and Physiology	1
2	What is Asthma?	9
3	Clinical Recognition	37
4	Complications of Asthma	47
5	Tests of Lung Function	53
6	Anti-asthma Drugs	75
7	Delivery Systems	91
8	The Management of Asthma and the Organization of Care	101
9	The Intangibles of Asthma Care: Aspects of Patient, Family and Professional Psychology in Practice	159
10	The Future	167
	Appendix 1: Relative monthly prescribing cost	171
	Appendix 2: Normal peak flow readings in adults and children	173
	Index	175

Acknowledgements

THE author would like to thank Greta Barnes with whom the concept of the practice nurse's role in the management of asthma was conceived and developed.

Thanks also to Val for her devoted secretarial work in typing the manuscript, and to Gillian Nineham and Kate Martin at Radcliffe Medical Press.

The publishers wish to thank Fisons for their financial support.

The author would like to dedicate this book to

Val, Dan and Ben.

Foreword

THE eminent Canadian physician and Regius Professor of Medicine in Oxford after whom the Unit in which I work is named – William Osler – thought asthma was a 'neurotic affection', and wrote in his classic text-book, 'death during the attack is unknown'. His treatment for attacks was chloroform, morphia and stramonium cigarettes, and he recommended potassium iodide as a preventative. Sixty years later when I was at medical school, MacLeans textbook of medical treatment acknowledged that, 'death is by no means rare'. He could offer adrenaline and ephedrine as well as cortisone to treat the attack: but sedation still featured prominently and there were no suggestions for preventing attacks.

Within the short space of just another fifteen years the face of asthma was changed beyond recognition by two novel approaches to treatment – prophylaxis and inhalers. The pioneering work of Altounyan on preventing allergen challenge from triggering asthma by the prior administration of disodium cromoglycate introduced the concept of prophylaxis. Frustration with the side effects of oral treatment led to the logical choice of the inhaled route for asthma therapy. The two were combined in the Intal Spincaps introduced in 1968. With the invention of the metered dose pressurized aerosol and its application first to bronchodilator therapy and then in 1972 to inhaled steroid therapy, the scene was set for all that has been done in asthma drug therapy since. More selective bronchodilators and minimally absorbed steroids have seen refinements rather than fundamental changes in treatment.

Important changes in the management of asthma of a quite different nature have taken place since these therapeutic advances, and are the motivation behind this book and Robert Pearson, its author. Certainly in these pages you will find an accurate account of the pathophysiology and cellular mechanisms that, as far as we can see, underlie the genesis of asthma. You will find too a detailed listing of the drug treatments that are available. But permeating its early pages and blossoming forth in the later chapters, you will find much more – an approach to management in the community beyond the whitewashed walls of the hospital, that is fundamentally a way of caring that is firmly orientated.

Neither of the major advances I have listed will work without that fundamental change in the doctor patient relationship from 'I tell: you do', to 'Together we plan, and understand', which is so much a part of the approach to asthma management set out in this book. Patients must understand their treatment in a more intimate and detailed way than they have ever had to do previously: they need education. This is not just imparting information, it is teaching skills as well. Inhaled drugs will not work if they are not taken properly: skills must be taught and their learning reinforced. In this respect Robert Pearson has had the unflagging support of his practice nurse partner, Greta Barnes. The Asthma Society Training Centre which they set up in Stratford-upon-Avon has proved beyond doubt the value of a collaborative approach to asthma care in practice. Countless nurses and others bear witness to the validity of the view of asthma expressed in these pages and have left their three day training course overwhelmingly better informed and fired with enthusiasm to carry the torch to their own health centres and practices.

The patient is seen to enter the picture not just as a recipient of drugs and goodwill, but as a partner in management, someone who will and can learn to adjust, anticipate, control their disease with reference back to the carers when needed, but more and more self managing. Partners too in what needs to be a concerted effort to find solutions to a disease that is still baffling in many respects. Asthma deaths and hospital admissions are rising. It seems as though overall prevalence is on the increase, but if so why? Can asthmatics themselves provide the answers? They have the disease. We should listen to them. Working in partnership with them to manage their disease and hear what they are saying may not just lead to better treatment of asthma but might hold the clue to some of its unanswered questions.

In reading these pages do not just learn the facts, you should know most of them anyway, but critically examine the management plan and ask how your approach matches up to the recommendations of the author. Above all take away something of the spirit that has inspired its writing.

Donald Lane
Oxford

Preface

THE purpose of this book is to bring the everyday management of asthma up-to-date, in order to take full advantage of the advances in our understanding of asthma and its treatment. There is still a wide gulf between what is possible and what is available to patients. There would have been no place for such a book twenty years ago, before the advent of today's most widely used therapeutic agents – specific $beta_2$-agonist bronchodilators, sodium cromoglycate, inhaled corticosteroids, nedocromil sodium and long acting preparations of theophylline.

To accommodate these new therapeutic agents it has been necessary to adopt an anticipatory approach to much asthma management. 'Medical Micawberism' – waiting for problems to occur and responding to them, is no longer either appropriate or acceptable. Anticipatory care takes a good deal more time and is discussed in the section on the organization of care, which introduces the concept of making greater use of specially trained nurses in order to create the additional practice time which becomes necessary.

However good the organization might be, it cannot compensate for a basic lack of understanding of asthma itself. The major part of the book sets out to relate the bronchi and their linings to the remainder of the respiratory tract. The definition, prevalence and impact of asthma are examined and the pathophysiology is related to symptoms. Emphasis is placed on the need to take a full clinical history and to include some type of objective measurement of airflow limitation in the overall assessment of each patient. The aim of therapy is to encourage a normal lifestyle and to prevent long term complications and the progression to irreversible airflow limitation. The morbidity and mortality of asthma are still considerably greater than should be the case if available therapy were properly applied.

It is essential that the practitioner understands that asthma is not synonymous with bronchoconstriction, but may also include the narrowing of airways due to mucosal oedema and mucus production. Another very relevant feature is bronchial hyperreactivity or hyperresponsiveness, itself the result of bronchial inflammation which leaves the bronchial smooth muscle very sensitive to minor stimuli or trigger factors, such as cold air or exercise.

Treatment must be planned to be appropriate to the occasion and in proportion to the severity of the asthma – it must be matched to the individual asthma sufferer. We must consider the types of drug that are indicated, and how they will be administered, bearing in mind the patient's likely compliance with one's advice and prescriptions.

So far I have emphasized the role of the doctor or nurse and the need for their continuing education. However, we must not forget the patient who has to live with the asthma and who must be involved in the thinking behind his or her treatment and its rationale. Doctors and patients may need to overcome a steroid phobia, but this is not to be looked upon as a *carte blanche* for the irresponsible overuse of corticosteroids. Whatever treatment is prescribed, it is mandatory to reassess the patient's response and need for that treatment. Severe asthma should be treated energetically and any maintenance therapy should be at the minimum effective level to minimize side effects.

I have written this book from the viewpoint of a committed, busy general practitioner. My interests do not lie solely in the field of asthma care but I do feel that the only practical place for most asthma care is in the setting of general practice. The necessary expertise is increasing, overall standards of care are slowly improving, but there is a long way to go before we achieve a uniform level. Different members of the primary care team have different roles to play, but family medicine must respond to the satisfiable needs of our patients and must not be found wanting.

We are all conscious of the financial implications of the care we offer, but we need to look beyond the cost of prescribed medication. At current UK prices, the cost of a typical year's inhaled preventive therapy, taken by aerosol inhaler is less than one day's stay in a district general hospital. A year's supply of dry powder preparations may be equivalent to two days in hospital. Compare this with the cost of an average stay in hospital which follows a severe exacerbation of asthma – often up to two or three weeks, to overcome the period of instability which may occur after a severe episode of asthma – one patient's stay might pay for the preventive therapy of twenty or more patients for a whole year! Such equations may be all too easily overlooked.

While I have tried to throw some light on a simplified approach to the pathophysiological events surrounding asthma, this field is highly complex, occasionally contradictary, but always moving forward at an exciting pace. The book is based broadly on my own practice, which I believe to be representative of asthma management in the United Kingdom.

Robert Pearson
December, 1989

1 Anatomy and Physiology

Similar lining throughout respiratory tract – Bronchial mucosa, submucosa, smooth muscle – Vagal innervation – Beta-adrenergic receptors – Ventilation and perfusion – Control of respiration

Respiration is the process whereby cells and organisms obtain energy. For the purposes of study, it can be divided into internal and external respiration. In this book, we will consider only external respiration which involves:

1 the physical act of breathing;
2 gaseous exchange: oxygen is taken up from the inspired air in the alveoli in exchange for carbon dioxide which is transported in the blood flowing through the pulmonary capillaries.

Structurally, the respiratory system may be divided into:

1 the upper respiratory tract;
2 the lower respiratory tract.

Upper respiratory tract

The upper respiratory tract comprises the nose (including the paranasal sinuses), the pharynx and the larynx, and serves many important functions:

- heat exchange, to warm inspired air;
- humidification, to moisten inspired air;
- filtration, to trap dust and particulate matter suspended in inspired air;
- sense of smell (olfactory organs);
- speech (larynx).

The oropharynx (Fig. 1.1, *see* overleaf), like the mouth and oesophagus, is lined with stratified squamous epithelium, similar to that of the epidermis. The remainder of the upper respiratory tract is lined with a mucus-secreting, ciliated columnar or pseudostratified epithelium. The cilia have a cleansing function and propel mucus, laden with particles, towards the pharynx, where it is swallowed. The mucoid secretions also protect these sensitive linings by preventing them from drying out.

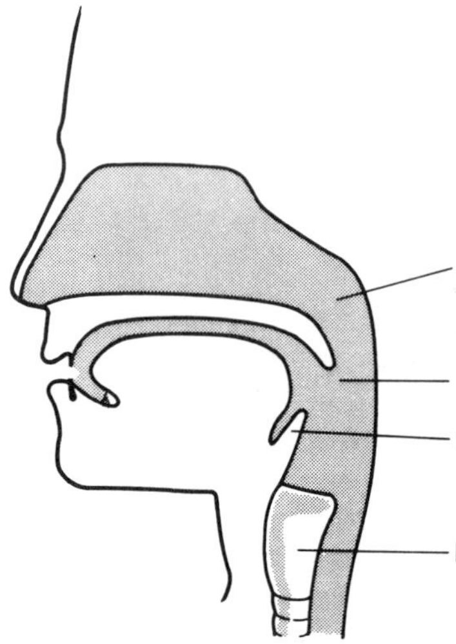

Figure 1.1 Upper respiratory tract.

The linings of the upper respiratory tract are vulnerable to viral infections, colonization by bacteria, the effects of fumes, inhalation of allergens and changes in environmental temperature and humidity. Attack by any of these factors may lead to acute or chronic inflammatory processes, with swelling of the mucosae, increased or altered secretions and obstruction to the natural drainage of secretions from the nasal passages and sinuses. Inflammation will profoundly affect the normal functions of the upper respiratory tract which may have secondary effects on the lower respiratory tract—air might bypass the nasal airways, or a cough may develop with aspiration from the overspill and drainage of fluid from the sinuses, particularly with postural changes.

Lower respiratory tract

The lower respiratory tract comprises the trachea, the bronchi and the lungs. The trachea is a fairly rigid tube passing down from the larynx; it divides at its lower end into right and left main bronchi (Fig. 1.2). It owes its rigidity to the C- or Y-shaped cartilaginous rings in its walls, although its posterior wall is composed only of smooth muscle. Cartilage rings or plates, interspersed with bundles of smooth muscle fibres, continue down the dividing bronchi until the bronchioles reach a diameter of only 1 mm. Like the upper respiratory tract, the trachea and bronchi share a continuous ciliated pseudostratified columnar epithelium containing numerous mucus-secreting goblet cells and small submucosal glands.

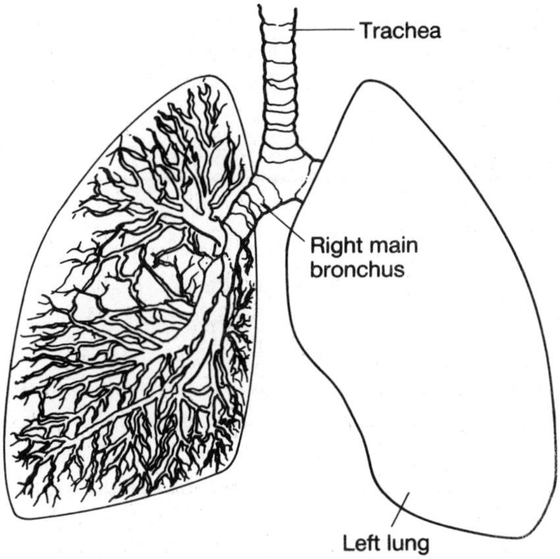

Figure 1.2 Representational diagram of lower respiratory tract.

The structure of the bronchi and bronchioles is central to our understanding of asthma and its therapy. In the course of over 20 repeated divisions, the bronchial tree descends from primary to secondary bronchi, to bronchioles, terminal bronchioles, respiratory bronchioles, alveolar ducts and sacs and finally to the alveoli. At the level of the respiratory bronchiole (a diameter of <0.5 mm), the mucosa no longer contains goblet cells and the columnar cells are low cuboidal and do not have cilia; the wall contains a network of elastic fibres and smooth muscle cells. The respiratory bronchioles give way to alveolar ducts and increasing numbers of alveoli; the latter resemble a hollow, air-containing honeycomb, and the alveolar walls are covered in a thin capillary network (Fig. 1.3). Air is

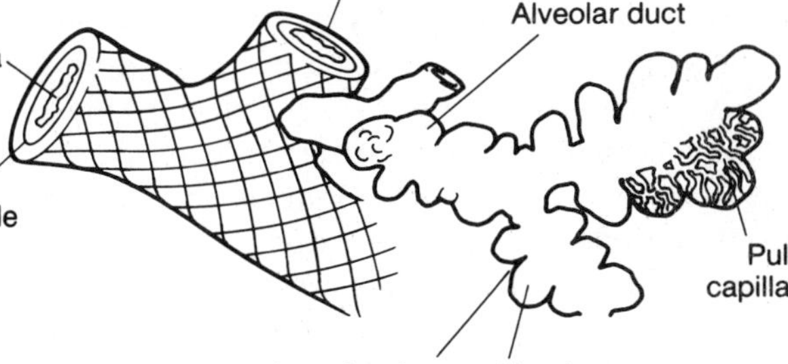

Figure 1.3 Structure of bronchi and bronchioles.

separated from the blood by flat alveolar cells, a basement membrane and the capillary endothelium. This arrangement maximizes the surface area available for the rapid exchange of oxygen and carbon dioxide between alveolar air and the blood.

During development, the bronchial tree is fully developed by the sixteenth week of intrauterine life; however, the alveoli continue to increase in number until the age of 8 years.

The simple subdivisions of the bronchial wall are shown in cross-section in Fig. 1.4 (a). More cellular detail is given in Fig. 1.4 (b). The mucosa, submucosa and circular/spiral smooth muscle coat all have a part to play in the pathogenesis of asthma, as will be explained later (*see* p. 15).

The goblet cells and submucosal glands receive vagal innervation, which is part of the cholinergic parasympathetic nervous system. The smooth muscle cells are also stimulated to contract by vagal nerve endings. Although there is sympathetic innervation to the pulmonary vasculature, it is thought that the adrenergic responses of the smooth muscle cells of the bronchi and bronchioles are mediated by circulating catecholamines, such as adrenaline. Stimulation of the beta-adrenergic receptors leads to smooth muscle relaxation.

The following sensory receptors are found in the lungs:

1 irritant receptors, lying between the epithelial cells, which characteristically lead to coughing, hyperventilation and perhaps vagally-mediated smooth muscle contraction;
2 stretch receptors, positioned between the smooth muscle cells, which respond to lung inflation.

In normal lungs, the resting control of the diameter of the airways appears to be predominantly vagal, as judged by the reduction in airflow resistance that occurs after the administration of atropine, an anticholinergic agent. When beta-adrenergic blockers are administered, the increase in resistance to flow is not consistent, suggesting that under normal conditions the sympathetic system plays little part in regulating bronchial tone.

In the lungs of an asthma sufferer, there is a normal response to cholinergic blockade. However, beta-adrenergic blockers are likely to increase airflow resistance, perhaps by reducing the increased resting sympathetic tone, which may be necessary to counteract other factors that tend to increase airways resistance. A likely mechanism of action is the blockade of beta-adrenoceptors to the effects of circulating catecholamines.

In the lungs, as in the gut, there is a network of non-cholinergic, non-adrenergic nerve fibres which produce neuropeptides; their role in normal lungs and in the pathogenesis of asthma is not known.

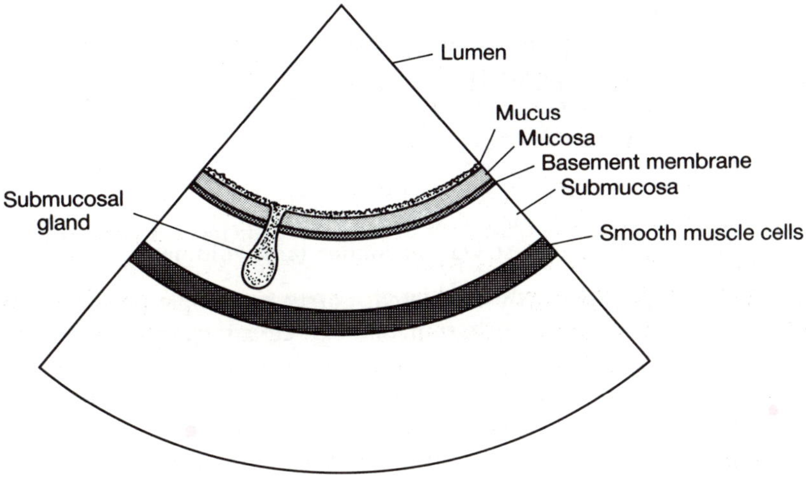

Figure 1.4 (a) Cross-section to show the subdivisions of the bronchial wall.

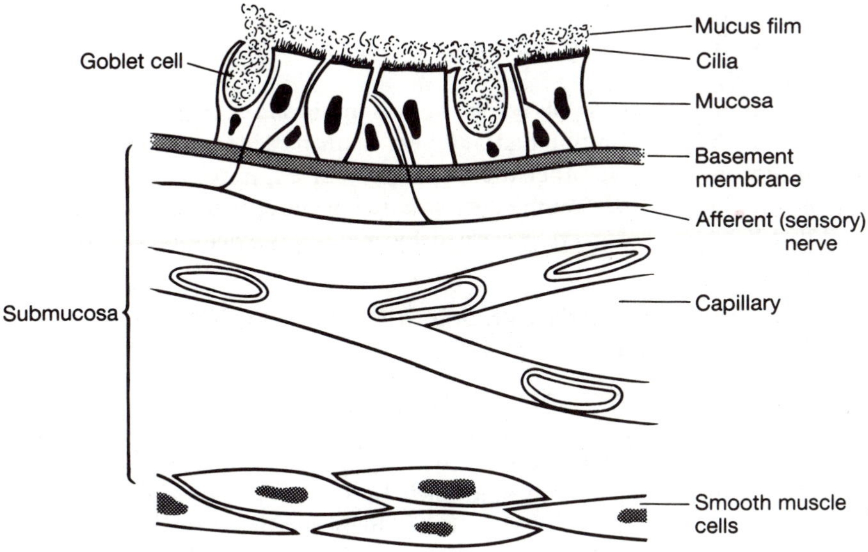

Figure 1.4 (b) Cellular detail of bronchial wall.

Control of breathing

Ventilation of the lungs has two phases: breathing in and breathing out. Ventilation is the result of the automatic rhythmic contractions of the respiratory muscles—the diaphragm and the intercostals.

The inspiratory muscles must overcome:

1 the resistance to airflow within the airways;
2 the intrinsic elasticity of the alveolar walls;
3 the elasticity of the chest wall at higher lung volumes.

The lungs are not uniformly ventilated, partly for simple physical reasons and partly because the distribution of inspired air changes according to the depth of the breath. At low lung volumes, the inspired air travels preferentially to the apices; as the lung volume rises, the air increasingly enters the bases. When respiratory demands are increased or there is any restriction of airflow, accessory muscles such as the sternomastoids are used to expand the upper chest.

Relaxed expiration depends upon the elastic recoil of the lungs, especially at full inflation. However, during forced expiration, pleural pressure becomes positive and assists the expiratory process, although any increase in expiratory flow is limited by those same forces causing a parallel compression of the airways.

Pulmonary blood flow is not uniform: there is a gradient of increasing flow from the apices down to the bases which is largely due to the effects of gravity. Thus, both ventilation and perfusion are greater at the lung bases.

The rhythmic nature of respiration is maintained by two groups of neurons in the medulla oblongata. These neurons send out impulses to the spinal motoneurons of either the inspiratory or expiratory muscles—those for the diaphragm, for example, are situated at the spinal level C5. The rate and depth of breathing are governed by medullary chemoreceptors which are sensitive to:

1 the carbon dioxide concentration of the blood (pCO_2);
2 the acidity or pH of the blood.

Rising pCO_2 or concentrations of acidic metabolites, such as lactate, will stimulate breathing, e.g. in diabetic ketoacidosis, renal failure or after exercise. A reduced pCO_2 lessens the respiratory drive. This explains the phenomenon of being able to hold one's breath for longer after a period of hyperventilation. A back-up system of chemoreceptors which respond to falls in the oxygen concentration in the arterial blood (pO_2) is to be found in the aortic and carotid bodies.

The lungs have an immense reserve capacity. A typical minute-volume of 7.5 litres of air (15 breaths/minute with a tidal volume of 500 ml) might rise by tenfold during vigorous exercise. Naturally, pulmonary blood flow will increase proportionately.

Approximately 140 ml of each breath is required to flush out the airways before the alveoli are reached—this is known as the anatomical dead space. The concept of dead space may seem to be unimportant when considering normal lungs, but it assumes considerable significance in the presence of a restricted tidal volume, especially when inhaled therapy is being used.

Summary

1 The upper and lower respiratory tracts interreact and have a common lining which may behave similarly.
2 A knowledge of the structure and behaviour of the bronchi and bronchioles is central to the understanding of asthma.
3 The distribution of air and blood within the lungs is sensitively matched and the balance is easily upset by malfunction of either ventilation, e.g. asthma or perfusion.

2 What is Asthma?

Variable resistance to airflow – A syndrome, not a single entity – Extrinsic, intrinsic, secondary and occupational – Atopy – IgE – Allergen – Mast cells – Type I, immediate hypersensitivity – Mediators – Smooth muscle contraction – Mucus hypersecretion – Mucosal oedema – Bronchial inflammation and hyperreactivity – Early asthmatic response – Late asthmatic response – Chemotactic factors – Eosinophils – Characteristic sputum – Enables rational approach to therapy – Current prevalence five per cent – Under-diagnosis – Is prevalence increasing? Ethnic and geographical differences – Hidden morbidity – 'Morning dip' – Preventable mortality – Poor patient education – Poor follow up – Insufficient prophylaxis – Underestimated severity – Trigger factors (infection, allergy, exercise, emotion, aspirin, beta-blockers, acid reflux, menstrual)

Definition

I have chosen Scadding's (1983) definition because it is clearer than many others:

> 'Asthma is a disease characterized by wide variations over short periods of time, in resistance to flow in intrapulmonary airways.'

These variations may appear to be spontaneous or to be precipitated by one of many factors, including therapy. Resistance to airflow may be chronically increased with superimposed exacerbations, or it may be normal between acute attacks.

The principal problem in defining asthma is that it is not a single disease entity. In practice, it is a disorder of function; it is a syndrome; it is the final common pathway of several pathological processes. Although no definition can be all-encompassing, it must be capable of undergoing expansion and development without losing its essential meaning.

Some degree of confusion surrounds the word 'asthma' and the explanation lies in semantics. The word asthma can be used in two different senses:

1 to describe the ongoing tendency to suffer from asthma in the past, currently or in the future;
2 to describe an acute event, with a sudden rise in airways resistance.

The definition of asthma may be very different from the conception of the condition held by GPs, nurses and the public. Conceptions will vary and may be erroneous, based upon ignorance and misinformation. All may agree that asthma is characterized by wheezing and breathlessness, but individual judgements may be clouded by prejudices associated with 'nervous asthma', which are still prevalent. Thus, whatever the true cause of the asthma, the onus is placed upon the shoulders of the sufferer.

It is impossible within the confines of an academic definition to convey the meaning of asthma, as experienced by an asthma sufferer but asthma can be appreciated at two levels.

1 The automatic physiological response to dysfunction in the pulmonary airways during which respiratory effort is increased and some degree of hyperventilation occurs; the response of the sympathetic nervous system is very restrained compared with its response to other threatening situations, such as myocardial infarction.
2 The subjective realization on the part of the sufferer that breathing is becoming more difficult and leading to physical restriction and the inability to respond normally to any additional energy expenditure. Indeed asthmatics may find it difficult to utter anything more than staccato words, thus severely reducing their ability to communicate at a time when it is imperative to do so.

Classification

Any current classification of asthma is only of limited value. Previously it was popular to classify the condition as being either intrinsic or extrinsic. Extrinsic asthma is characteristically associated with a reaction to an outside agent and, typically, evidence of allergic reactions may be apparent, whereas with intrinsic asthma, allergic reactions are absent. Although I have retained this basic division, I have also included two further categories – secondary and occupational asthma. Exercise-induced asthma is sometimes treated as a separate category, but it is most conveniently considered as a facet of any other 'types' of asthma.

Extrinsic asthma

- Sufferers are more likely to show a family history of asthma.
- Most sufferers are atopic, which means that they exhibit skin reactions when tested with appropriate allergens.
- There is a strong association with hay fever, eczema, allergic rhinitis and urticaria.
- Symptoms commonly start in childhood.
- Symptoms are often episodic and there may be long periods of remission.

Intrinsic asthma

- There is an absence of demonstrable hypersensitivity reactions.
- Sufferers develop asthma during or after middle age.
- Symptoms are more likely to be persistent.
- Symptoms may respond only to treatment with corticosteroids.
- There may be an interesting association with aspirin sensitivity and nasal polyps.

Secondary asthma

- Occasionally an asthma syndrome occurs in association with chronic lung diseases, such as sarcoidosis and bronchiectasis.
- Specific treatment of the primary disorder may reduce symptoms but treatment of the asthma component is often necessary.
- As asthma is a common disorder, some individuals might have displayed asthmatic symptoms in the absence of this other condition but in other sufferers it may be a truly secondary phenomenon.

Occupational asthma

- Some asthma is related solely to the working environment of the sufferer and may resolve after removal or avoidance of the cause.
- The proportion of workers affected and the severity of the asthma are related to the agent concerned, the level of exposure and the degree of individual susceptibility.
- Some industrial substances give rise to symptoms through hypersensitivity reactions, but other substances may behave as chemical inducers.
- Symptoms are typically worse during the working week and may diminish or disappear during weekends or absence from work.
- The severity of the asthma may worsen progressively with repeated, prolonged exposure.
- Apart from separation from the injurious agent, occupational asthma is treated by conventional means.

- Substances recognized in the United Kingdom for industrial compensation after appropriate verification are:

  platinum salts
  isocyanates
  epoxy resins
  colophony fumes
  proteolytic enzymes
  grain or flour dust
  laboratory animals and insects
  cimetidine
  wood dust
  ispaghula
  castor bean dust
  ipecacuanha
  azo dicarbonamide

Asthma and atopy

Atopy is a constitutional tendency in certain persons to develop immediate or Type I hypersensitivity reactions such as with asthma or hay fever. It is also the name applied to the local reaction of the skin when an allergen is applied to it, by skin-prick for example. Hypersensitivity reactions are inappropriate responses of the immune system, the results of which are injurious to the host. Four types of hypersensitivity reaction are recognized but Type I is the one that concerns us here.

Type I hypersensitivity reactions are mediated by immunoglobulin E (IgE) antibody, which is normally produced in response to parasitic infections.

To demonstrate an atopic manifestation by a skin test requires:

1 a host capable of making inappropriate amounts of IgE antibody against everyday substances;
2 the presence of an antigen or 'allergen';
3 attachment of the specific IgE molecules to the surface of tissue mast cells at the site of the skin test.

This interaction between mast cells, IgE and the allergen is detrimental to the host. The natural reaction may occur in any of the body's tissues—the exact site governs the nature of the manifestation (Fig. 2.1). The Type I hypersensitivity reaction is an important link between these atopic phenomena and is one of the triggering mechanisms for asthma.

Asthma and allergy are not synonymous. The inheritance of asthma is complex, whereas atopy is transmitted as an autosomal dominant, which means that a carrier of this dominant gene has a one in two chance of passing it on to each child. Raised levels of IgE may be found in the cord blood at birth and indicate future atopy. However, the appearance of any atopic manifestations is dependent upon the host and upon environmental factors. The development of atopic symptoms may be explained by changes in the permeability of gastrointestinal and respiratory mucous membranes (cigarette

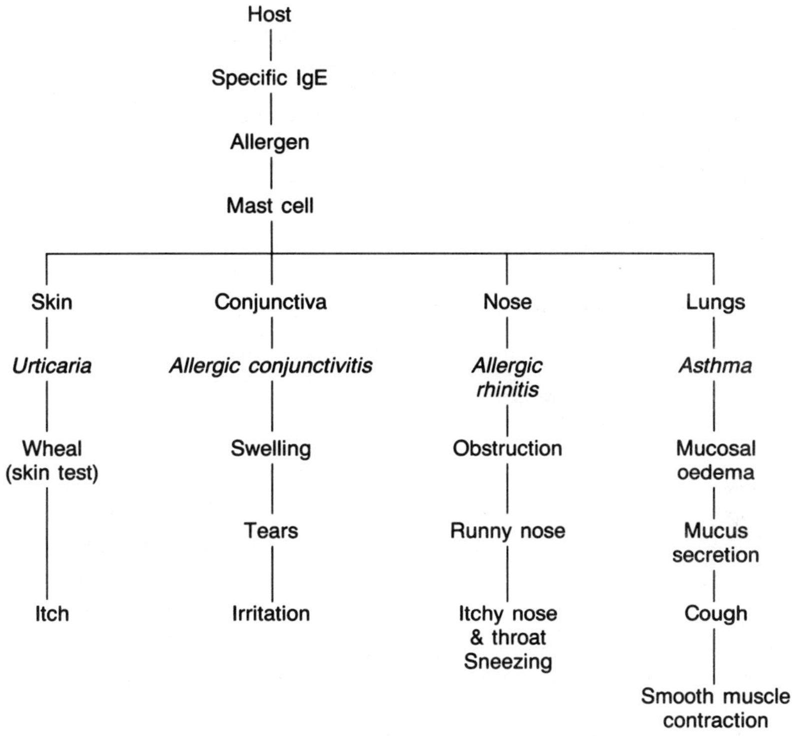

Figure 2.1 Everyday manifestations of Type I hypersensitivity reactions.

smokers have higher levels of IgE), a deficiency of neutralizing antibodies in the mucosae or a failure to suppress the inappropriate production of IgE. IgE is produced by lymphocytes in the respiratory and gastrointestinal submucosae and their associated lymph nodes, and its production is normally a controlled process.

Mast cells are found throughout the body but particularly in association with respiratory and gastrointestinal mucous membranes. They are related to the basophil cell of the granulocyte series. The mast cell membrane is able to fix specific IgE molecules which are then free to attach to antigen or allergen molecules. If an allergen bridges between two IgE molecules, degranulation of the mast cell follows (Fig. 2.2, *see* overleaf), thereby releasing mediators into the surrounding tissue fluids. In addition to the mediators, chemotactic factors are present which attract more mast cells, a situation well recognized in the allergic rhinitis of hay fever. Mediators are responsible for the clinical picture seen wherever a natural Type I hypersensitivity reaction takes place (*see* Fig. 2.1). The pattern of symptoms is as follows: oedema occurs as a result of increased capillary permeability;

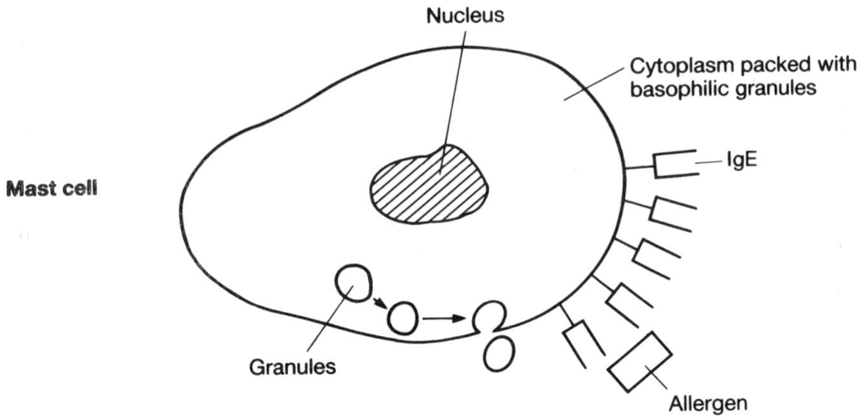

Figure 2.2 Mast cell.

glandular secretions increase; and irritation causes itching, sneezing or coughing. An additional element in asthma is that smooth muscle cells in the bronchial and bronchiolar walls also respond to these mediators by contracting.

Pathophysiology

Clinically, asthma is characterized by:

1 breathlessness;
2 wheeze;
3 chest tightness;
4 cough, either dry or productive.

These symptoms may be precipitated by many factors, for example exercise, or they may occur apparently spontaneously, for instance in the early hours of the morning, the so-called 'morning dip'. These diverse symptoms may have in common a triad of pathological features, although all three may not necessarily occur together (Fig. 2.3):

1 contraction of bronchial and bronchiolar smooth muscle, which leads to a rapid increase in airflow resistance within the bronchi and bronchioles, but which is rapidly reversed by inhaled $beta_2$-agonists (bronchodilators);
2 increased secretion of bronchial mucus;
3 oedema of the bronchial mucosa.

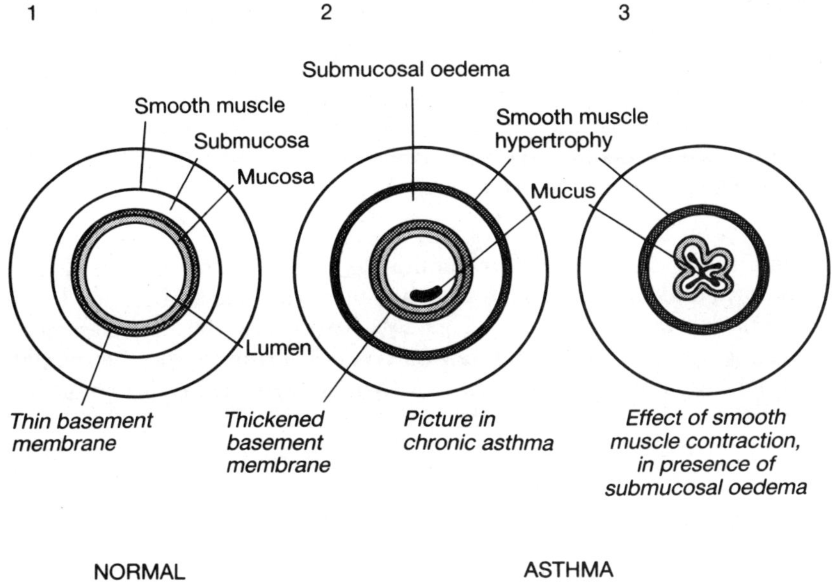

Figure 2.3 Triad of pathological features.

Increased secretion of bronchial mucus and oedema of the bronchial mucosa are associated with a slower, progressive increase in resistance to airflow, which is more persistent than that due to smooth muscle contraction and which can be reversed therapeutically only by systemic corticosteroids. Associated with all three features is bronchial hyperreactivity or hyperresponsiveness, the result of a persistent inflammatory process in the bronchial mucosa and submucosa. The effect is to lower the individual's threshold of responsiveness to the many trigger factors for asthma, leading to an increase in airways resistance.

The asthmatic bronchi show varying degrees of smooth muscle hypertrophy, thickening of the basement membrane and oedema of the submucosa. The degree of obstruction caused by the same extent of smooth muscle contraction will depend upon the current level of submucosal oedema—the greater the oedema, the greater the obstruction with superimposed smooth muscle spasm (*see* Fig. 2.3). There may be no underlying submucosal oedema and little or no evidence of any inflammatory process.

The temptation to explain the different elements of asthma, as if one simple process linked them together, must be resisted. As more information about the different mechanisms involved in asthma is obtained, all the evidence indicates that there are several parallel or converging processes which may be responsible for the individual clinical picture. Having said this, until the intricacies of the different types of asthma are understood, some form of working model is necessary. The model I shall use is an amalgam of the picture seen in allergen-provoked asthma in man and that observed in animal models.

Let us envisage an atopic asthmatic, who is sensitive to a particular allergen to which he or she is about to be exposed for a 5-minute period. The peak expiratory flow rate (PEFR) has already been measured and recordings will be taken every 5 or 10 minutes over the next few hours. Two patterns of response may occur.

1 In 50% of asthmatics, there will be only an 'early asthmatic response' with rapid onset of airflow limitation which reaches its peak by 30 minutes and then lessens until it has been restored to baseline by 2 – 3 hours, leaving no sequelae (Fig. 2.4). Its rapid onset, its relatively fast decline and the fact that it can be reversed promptly by the inhalation of beta$_2$-agonists, clearly indicates that this response is due to bronchial and bronchiolar smooth muscle contraction.
2 The remaining 50% of asthmatics display a 'dual response', in which the early asthmatic response is followed by the 'late asthmatic response', when, shortly after the return to baseline, at 3 – 4 hours there is again the onset of progressive airflow limitation, with a falling PEFR, which reaches its peak after about 8 – 12 hours from initial exposure, again regaining baseline by 24 hours (Fig. 2.4). It is possible to demonstrate enhanced bronchial hyperreactivity for up to 3 – 4 weeks after a single exposure. The inhalation of beta$_2$-agonists has only a marginal effect upon the increased airflow limitation suggesting that this is predominantly a submucosal and mucosal problem.

The differences between the clinical pictures of the early and dual asthmatic responses can be illustrated anecdotally (*see* page 18).

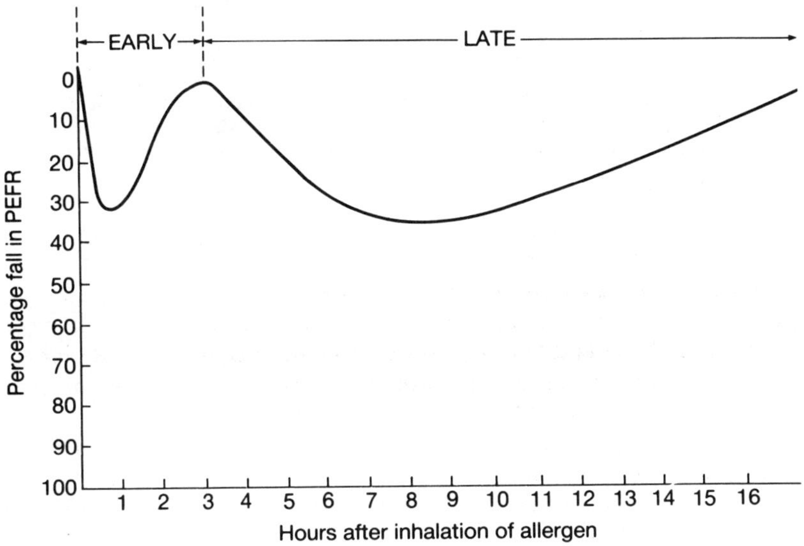

Figure 2.4 Changes in PEFR after brief inhalation of allergen – early and late asthmatic responses.

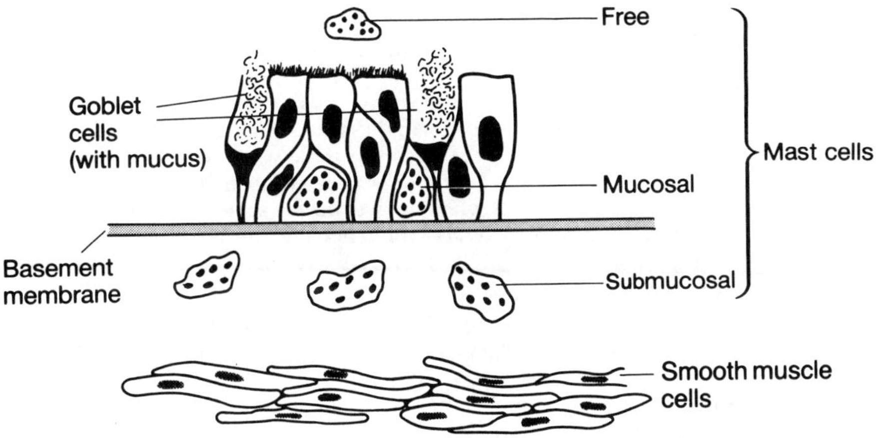

Figure 2.5 Bronchus in early asthmatic responses.

Thomas and Alexander Taylor are brothers aged 8 and 10 years respectively. They come from a strongly atopic family and they are both asthmatic. One Saturday, at lunchtime, they leave home to visit their grandmother who is widowed and has two cats and a dog. Thomas and Alexander love her pets, but at a price!

Shortly after they arrive, both boys develop itchy eyes, which they cannot resist rubbing and they start to sniff and to sneeze; soon they begin to cough and wheeze. Fortunately, mother is armed with a Rotahaler and the boys both take a salbutamol rotacap, with rapid relief of their asthmatic symptoms. They resume their play but, although Thomas remains well, by teatime Alexander is again beginning to cough and wheeze a little and despite taking more salbutamol his coughing and wheezing increase progressively. By early evening, Thomas again develops a wheeze which is relieved by salbutamol, but Alexander is now quite distressed. Initially restless, he is quiet and sitting at table, shoulders hunched, with a tight cough and difficult wheezy breathing. Salbutamol offers him the most marginal relief and it is decided to go home.

On the way home, Thomas is free of symptoms but is concerned about his brother who is not at all well. Although Thomas goes straight to bed and has a good night's sleep, Alexander remains downstairs with his parents as he cannot comfortably lie down, due to his dyspnoea. Finally, he goes to bed, where tiredness overcomes him and he falls asleep, propped up with several pillows. Sleep is fitful but Alexander's asthma reaches the peak of its severity in the early hours of the morning, his parents spending most of the night in his room, giving him his salbutamol Rotacaps with little effect, at least partly because he is unable to take a well co-ordinated suck. His asthma is certainly bad enough to warrant a night call to their doctor.

By breakfast time on Sunday, when Thomas is bright and lively, Alexander is still coughing and wheezing but less than during the night and as the day progresses he slowly improves, and with the removal of the allergic triggers his clinical asthma settles. The least exertion makes him breathless and wheezy, but this responds to salbutamol. He is quite comfortable when he goes to bed but he starts to cough and wakes up wheezing in the early hours. Again salbutamol helps him but he still has a cough when he gets up for school on Monday and it will be some days before his exercise tolerance and sleep pattern return to normal, due to persistent bronchial hyperreactivity.

There is a big difference between these two clinical pictures. Interestingly, although Thomas responded well to salbutamol, he would have been equally well protected by the prophylactic use of sodium cromoglycate. While Alexander gained initial relief from salbutamol, the relief lessened as the mucosal element of the late response became apparent. Again, he would have benefited from the prophylactic use of sodium cromoglycate before they left home to visit their grandmother. The combined use of inhaled salbutamol and beclomethasone would have had a similar protective effect.

How can we explain these events? To gain some insight we must return to the Type I hypersensitivity reaction. The inhaled allergen must have the right dimensions to reach the peripheral bronchi and bronchioles where the most telling reactions take place. Picture the bronchiolar wall at the moment of exposure (Fig. 2.5) with a few mast cells scattered in the submucosa, perhaps lying between epithelial cells and in the lumen. Molecules of IgE of appropriate specificity are attached to the surface membranes of the mast cells. Challenge with the allergen, whether inhaled or systemic, allows the allergen molecule to bridge between the two IgE molecules. This leads to two events:

1 degranulation of the mast cells, with the release of preformed mediators from within the granules;
2 production of membrane-derived mediators.

It has long been recognized that histamine is released from mast cell granules, but we now know of other substances that are also released, for example, a neutrophil chemotactic factor, an eosinophil chemotactic factor and possibly a basophil chemotactic factor. Histamine, by its own direct action, can cause intense bronchoconstriction which can be blocked by antihistamines, but this has little effect upon the development of the early asthmatic response. It is difficult to determine the roles of all these different agents and undue emphasis should not be placed on any one factor in the underlying mechanism.

The membrane-derived mediators are formed from phospholipids in the cell membrane, through the action of an enzyme, phospholipase A_2, which produces arachidonic acid. Arachidonic acid may then follow one of two pathways:

1 the cyclo-oxygenase pathway to form prostaglandins, prostacyclin and thromboxanes;
2 the lipoxygenase pathway which results in the production of leukotrienes, some of which were corporately identified as slow-reacting substance of anaphylaxis (SRS-A).

Histamine, some prostaglandins and leukotrienes can induce smooth muscle spasm, mucus production, increased vascular permeability and mucosal oedema; thromboxanes can cause bronchial hyperreactivity. The problem is fitting the known mediators to the known clinical picture in both early and late asthmatic responses.

The precise events leading to the late response are not known. Previously, a Type III or delayed hypersensitivity reaction was thought to play a part, but it now seems more likely that the late response follows mast cell activation, perhaps in relation to higher levels of IgE. Certainly, the evidence from biopsies suggests that, after the initial insult to the mast cells, there is a progressive influx, first of neutrophils then of eosinophils, presumably attracted by appropriate chemotactic factors. The leucocytes first adhere to capillary walls then enter the submucosa, gradually migrating towards the smooth muscle cells and the epithelium. Eosinophils can reduce mast cell activity and can also produce mediators which are more damaging than those released from the mast cells. The late phase probably involves mast cell reactivation, to which the membrane-derived mediators contribute, their action being longer lasting than that of histamine. Macrophages, some with specific IgE attached, start to influence events, perhaps by further activating and degranulating the eosinophils. Eosinophils release major basic protein and eosinophil cationic protein both of which are cytotoxic to the bronchial epithelium, which may be shed, thereby exposing the interepithelial nerve endings (Fig. 2.6). Stimulation of these nerve endings may trigger vagal effects or even 'axon reflexes' during which antidromic impulses contribute to the inflammatory process.

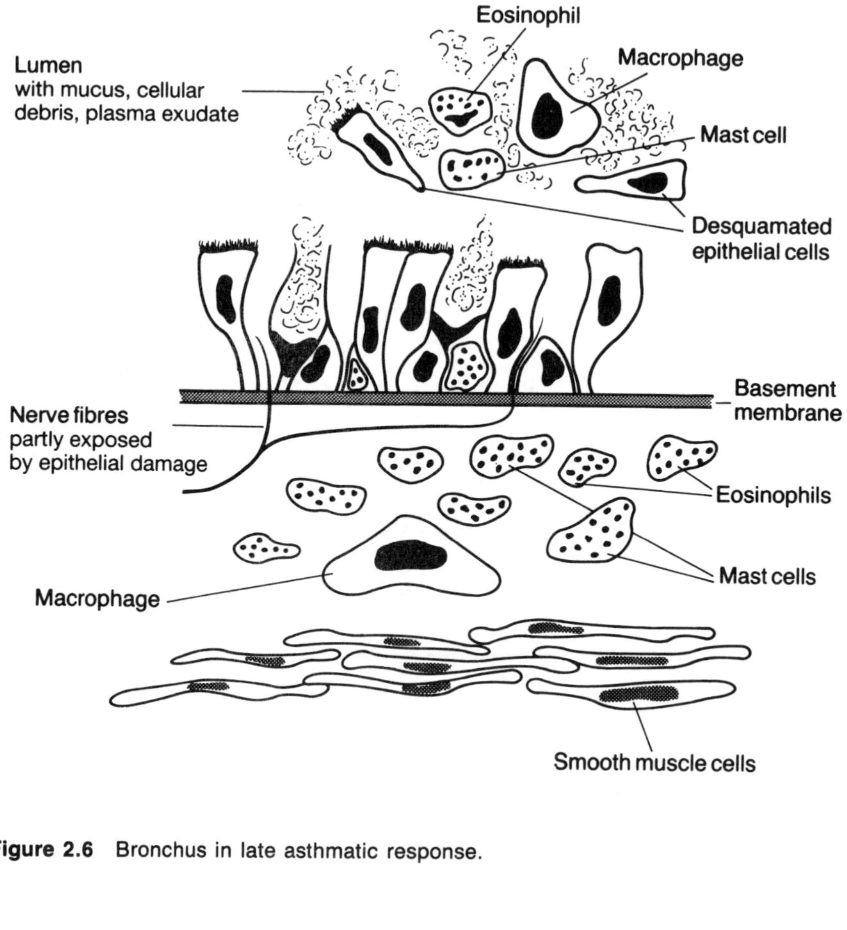

Figure 2.6 Bronchus in late asthmatic response.

In addition to the thromboxanes, platelet-activating factor (another product of granulocytic degranulation) is a potent stimulator of bronchial hyperreactivity. It may take very few cells or even residual bound mediators to maintain a background of bronchial hyperreactivity. Bronchial hyperreactivity can be assessed experimentally by measuring the increase in airways resistance in response to the inhalation of histamine or methacholine at progressively increasing concentrations. The greater the degree of hyperreactivity, the lower the concentration that provokes smooth muscle spasm. An arbitrary fall in PEFR or forced expiratory volume (FEV_1) of 20% is taken as significant.

The lumen of the bronchi will contain asthmatic sputum which is typically very sticky and almost rubbery. The complex nature of this sputum is shown in Fig. 2.6, with cellular elements in the form of eosinophils, mast cells, macrophages, damaged epithelial cells, plasma that has leaked from damaged capillaries, mucus secretions and Charcot–Leyden crystals derived from eosinophil cell membranes. The sputum may be so thick that it forms casts of the bronchioles and smaller bronchi. A simplified summary of these events is shown in Fig. 2.7, *see* overleaf.

Prolonged bronchial wall inflammation of this type will be damaging and may lead ultimately to irreversible airflow limitation.

The reasons for describing these mechanisms in some detail are:

1 to indicate the complexities of the situation which effectively rule out any simple solutions;
2 to introduce a rational approach to therapy by relating drug actions to the oversimplified picture of events in the early and late asthmatic responses. The basic responses to exercise are similar to the early asthmatic response and so treatment is as for the early response. This approach is summarized in Fig. 2.8, *see* page 23.

Prevalence

Part of the challenge that faces all of us who manage asthma in primary care stems from the fact that asthma is so common. In the United Kingdom, a commonly accepted figure for current prevalence is 5%, with a cumulative prevalence of 10 – 15% of population. Current prevalence refers to the number of sufferers within a defined period of study and cumulative prevalence includes all those who have ever suffered from the condition. In a typical practice of 10 000 patients, there will be approximately 500 current asthmatics, some of whom may not be recognized. In addition, there is a pool of 1000 potential sufferers who have had asthma in the past and who should be considered as being ‘asthmatic’ to avoid iatrogenic

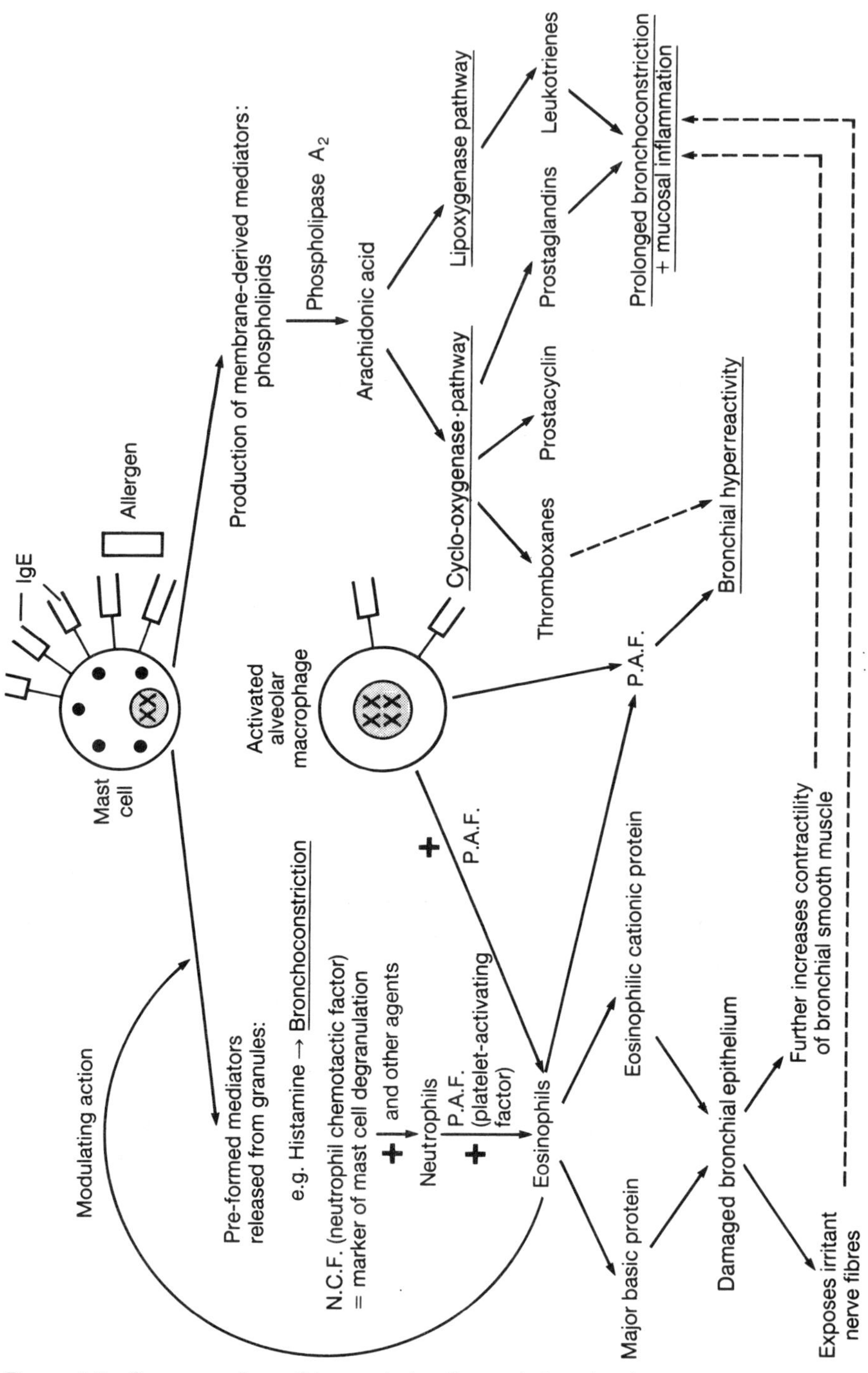

Figure 2.7 Summary of possible events in allergen-induced asthma.

	PREVENTION	TREATMENT
	Block by pre-treatment with:	Reverse with:
Early asthmatic response	Inhaled { $Beta_2$-agonist Sodium cromoglycate Nedocromil sodium	Inhaled $beta_2$-agonist
Late asthmatic response	Inhaled { Sodium cromoglycate Nedocromil sodium Corticosteroids	Systemic corticosteroids

Figure 2.8 Summary of a rational approach to early and late asthmatic responses.

problems, such as the prescription of beta-blocking drugs for example, whether for cardiovascular or ophthalmological purposes. It is estimated that there are 2.5 million current asthmatics in the United Kingdom.

At present, there is much discussion about whether asthma is becoming more common or whether its severity is changing. These questions are difficult to answer. Although the existence of many cases of asthma has always been undeniable, there are many asthmatics who have not been diagnosed as such, because, it is said, some doctors may not have wished to upset particular patients with the news. This approach was understandable when there was no effective treatment available, but there is no such excuse today. We have all seen patients and parents whose initial response, as soon as the word 'asthma' is used, is one of horror or despondence, seeing this as the beginning of a sedentary life for the sufferer, and one in which he or she will not be able to take part in active pursuits. To overcome this hurdle requires much explanation, a willingness to answer questions honestly and a preparedness to explore appropriate treatment with the patient, building up mutual trust and confidence with each consultation. The need for this degree of involvement may inhibit some doctors and may explain why there has been such a marked underdiagnosis and under-reporting of asthma. However, the failure to diagnose and name asthma almost guarantees incorrect, inadequate or inappropriate treatment, thereby maintaining a higher level of morbidity.

It is important to keep an open mind on the question of the changing prevalence of asthma. The increase in reported asthma may result from:

1 a *real* increase in prevalence due to some unidentified factor(s);
2 an *apparent* increase in prevalence due to an increase in numbers of cases diagnosed. This results from a greater understanding of asthma and the wide availability of effective therapeutic agents, which make recognition and diagnosis more worthwhile.

It is impossible to compare with any validity prevalence from before about 1970 with today's figures because circumstances and criteria are so different. For example, a diligent search within a single practice may double the number of asthmatic children recognized. Speight's studies on North Tyneside (Lee *et al.*, 1983; Speight *et al.*, 1983) were an epidemiological and clinical watershed in the management of asthma in terms of identifying prevalence, morbidity, underdiagnosis and under-treatment and in demonstrating the results of diagnosis and subsequent treatment. In a population of seven-year-olds, the recognized cumulative prevalence was 1.3%, but when diagnostic criteria laid down for the study were applied this figure rose to 11.1%.

The cumulative figures for our practice in Stratford-upon-Avon in 1987 are shown in Fig. 2.9. These confirm a striking preponderance of males, particularly in young patients. Prevalence is highest in the young, who represent a disproportionate fraction of the total current asthma sufferers. The very young are under-represented because only those who are clearly asthmatic are diagnosed when it is possible to identify the symptoms between bouts of respiratory viral infections. The cumulative adult prevalence will slowly increase as today's younger diagnosed asthmatics get older.

Female	**Age**	**No.**	**Asthma**	**%**
	0 – 6 yrs	291	9	3.1%
	7 – 14 yrs	406	45	11.1%
	14 – 21 yrs	487	33	6.8%
	Over 21 yrs	4078	213	5.2%
Male	**Age**	**No.**	**Asthma**	**%**
	0 – 6 yrs	282	24	8.5%
	7 – 14 yrs	440	74	16.8%
	14 – 21 yrs	502	62	12.4%
	Over 21 yrs	3485	234	6.7%
Overall by age	**Age**			**%**
	0 – 6 yrs			5.8%
	7 – 14 yrs			14.1%
	14 – 21 yrs			9.6%
	Over 21 yrs			5.9%
Overall by sex		Female = 5.7%	Male = 8.4%	

Total number of asthmatics = 7%
Practice population = 9971

Figure 2.9 Cumulative prevalence of asthma in author's practice, 1987.

I stated earlier that atopic manifestations depend upon a complex interplay between a changing host and a changing environment. This statement also applies to the symptoms of asthma. There are fascinating differences in prevalence not only between different ethnic groups in one geographical location but also within a single ethnic group that has been divided by migration. The reasons for these differences are complex. Some individual asthmatics are aware of seasonal variation and the effect on symptoms of different houses, workplaces, districts and countries. Every piece of information may further elucidate the mechanisms of asthma and the factors that govern it.

In this era of information technology, with ease of information storage and retrieval, it should be possible to follow population groups living in a particular area and to study prospectively the outcome in individual patients and groups, thus providing useful information about the epidemiology of asthma.

Morbidity and mortality

The symptoms of asthma cover a wide spectrum, ranging from those that are mild and intermittent, such that the sufferer may not be aware that they have the condition, to those that are severe and chronic, such that the sufferer is subject to potentially fatal exacerbations. Morbidity may be easy to identify in an individual but it is difficult to measure statistically in a population. For an individual, morbidity is a 'deficit in their quality of life'. To study morbidity we must assess such things as the number of days lost from school or work, the number of nights of broken sleep, the inability to take part in games, either occasionally or always. However, the resources required to do this are considerable.

Over 25% of the asthmatic children studied in North Tyneside had their level of physical activity restricted. The tale of the asthmatic goalkeeper, defender or score-keeper is quite true and will be encountered frequently. Absenteeism in the presence of poorly controlled asthma may be considerable; some of the North Tyneside seven-year-olds had lost over 50 school days in the year. Effective therapy reduced absenteeism by tenfold.

Nocturnal disturbances, i.e. waking up coughing and wheezing in the early hours of the morning—'the morning dip'—(*see* Fig. 5.2, p.58), represent broken or totally disrupted sleep, not just for the sufferer but for the whole household. The family's response will be a mixture of sympathy and resentment. Dream sleep (REM sleep) is associated with a 'dip' superimposed on the 'morning dip'. Apart from feeling physically tired in the daytime, the child will suffer additionally from disturbance to his or her growth pattern. This could be related to the fact that growth hormone is produced in bursts during REM sleep and during vigorous exercise. In addition to growth suppression, there may be delayed puberty and a postponed growth spurt, both of which may impose a considerable psychological burden upon any child within his or her peer group.

Underachievement breeds low expectations. Parents may only recognize the magnitude of the problem after the child has been on effective treatment for some time, which has led to an increase in exercise tolerance and a decrease in the time lost from school.

Adults, especially those within competitive labour markets, will be unwilling to absent themselves from work except in the most exceptional circumstances. Consequently, the value of figures for time lost from work due to asthma may be questionable. Younger sufferers have difficulty when participating in sporting activities, whereas older patients will experience problems in walking to the shops and even when doing the housework. Unfortunately, and sometimes to their ultimate cost, asthmatics suffer and tolerate too much without complaint—perhaps because they feel that nothing can be done to help them or because they have not been helped in the past when they should have been.

Morbidity from asthma may be considerable. Occasionally such morbidity is the sequel to asthma that is truly difficult to treat, but usually it is the result of asthma that has not been diagnosed or when appropriate treatment has not been given following diagnosis. In addition, in the United Kingdom, about 2000 patients are certified each year as having died from asthma, including about 50 children under 15 years of age. Investigations into asthma deaths have suggested that there were preventable factors in over 80% of cases, and treatment was usually deemed to have been too little, given too late.

Some hospital units have developed a self-admission policy for those patients who suffer from severe asthma that deteriorates rapidly. However, within hospitals, the best care will be received in thoracic units where all the staff are skilled in the care and monitoring of asthma. Problems are more likely to occur on general medical wards where skills may exist in other fields but not particularly in asthma. Even in hospital, some patients may not be recognized as suffering from asthma, but will be treated as having 'chest infections' or bronchitis.

The British Thoracic Association's confidential inquiry into asthma deaths in those aged between 15 and 64 years in the West Midlands and Mersey regions in 1979, yielded some disturbing information which led to the following conclusions and recommendations.

1 Diagnosis—in order to be treated effectively asthma must first be diagnosed.
2 Patient education of a basic type must be provided in order that the patient understands his or her asthma and its treatment.

3 Follow up is imperative in all asthmatics, especially in those with severe asthma who are more likely to suffer from severe exacerbations.
4 Prophylaxis—although inadequately used, it should be the mainstay of treatment rather than a reliance upon crisis remedies.
5 Deterioration—patients should know how to recognize deterioration and how to treat themselves with high-dose corticosteroids while seeking further medical assistance.
6 Emergency treatment—it is important that patients, relatives and doctors recognize severe asthma and institute appropriate treatment, perhaps with admission to hospital. For some patients early admission to hospital is mandatory, based upon experience on previous occasions. It must be stressed to some patients that their well-being is of prime importance and they must overcome their reluctance to call the GP.

It should be remembered that some of the patients most at risk are those with severe asthma who are beginning to respond to vigorous therapy. Their bronchi may become destabilized, and as the consistently high level of airflow resistance, which has been present for some time, lowers, the bronchi become highly hyperreactive. Death may occur during one of the sudden severe dips. This can happen in hospital or at home after discharge, at a time when peak flow monitoring is essential. In the presence of these severe swings the patient would be safer in hospital under the care of a respiratory physician.

If we apply the information already available to us we ought to be able to reduce the unnecessary morbidity of asthma and the preventable element of asthma mortality. Patients, doctors and nurses must collaborate in overcoming these problems—there is nothing to be gained from the three groups pulling, or being pulled, in different directions.

Asthma trigger factors

If we accept the concept of bronchial hyperreactivity we have to consider the role of different agents and events that might either promote hyperreactivity or behave as 'trigger factors' when another agent has caused the hyperreactivity. Often the route involved in triggering the asthma may be shared by different trigger factors. For example:

- infections;
- allergic reactions: (i) inhaled; (ii) ingested;
- exercise;
- laughing, hyperventilation, cold air;
- emotion—'psychological';
- non-specific irritants, e.g. cigarette smoke;
- aspirin and non-steroidal anti-inflammatory drugs;

- beta-blocking drugs;
- gastro-oesophageal reflux;
- menstrual factors.

Infections

Respiratory tract viruses, for example rhinoviruses, may cause virus-induced mucosal inflammation and associated bronchial hyperreactivity. The results of home monitoring in a 30-year-old man whose asthma prophylaxis was not quite adequate are shown in Fig. 2.10. He was recording his PEFR every third day. After the onset of a respiratory tract infection, his PEFR began to fall but there was still a good response to bronchodilator inhalation. However, the post-bronchodilator PEFR was always lower than it was before the infection intervened. Failure to dilate the bronchi to their previous level was due to mucosal oedema. In his case, recovery without any additional therapy took about 1 month. The time course of recovery will vary considerably between individuals.

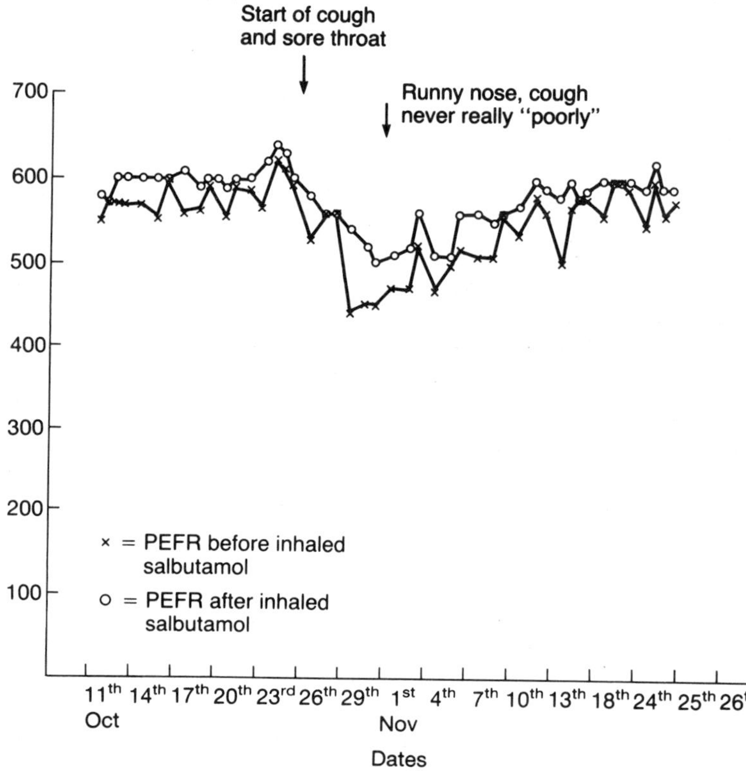

Figure 2.10 PEFR monitoring before and during a respiratory tract infection (readings on rising, lunchtime, teatime, bedtime).

Interestingly, some viruses may cause similar epithelial damage to that occurring with a severe late asthmatic response, resulting in the exposure of irritant nerve endings. This may explain why non-asthmatic subjects can suffer from bronchial hyperreactivity after some viral respiratory tract infections. The hyperreactivity lasts for about 2 months but is not usually of the same degree of severity as that seen in asthma.

Another point of interest is that *Haemophilus influenzae*, which is a common respiratory pathogen and opportunistic super-infecting organism, is capable of producing histamine. Thus, *Haemophilus* infections involve an additional potential trigger apart from the inflammatory process itself. This may have therapeutic implications for the treatment of asthma associated with infections, but it does not alter the basic rule that the asthma should be treated first. If the primary infection is viral, it is usually not amenable to specific treatment; however, if the infection is bacterial, antibiotics can be used in carefully judged situations.

In general, an appreciation of the mechanisms involved allows a more rational therapeutic approach. Thus, demonstrable bronchoconstriction will respond to beta$_2$-agonist bronchodilators, whereas mucosal problems and hyperreactivity must be treated in the usual way, with corticosteroids and inhaled prophylactic agents, respectively.

Allergic reactions

Allergic reactions are a common and potent trigger of the asthma process. So common, in fact, that the layman often equates the phenomena as being synonymous. This can give rise to problems in that some patients believe that asthma is potentially avoidable. This may sometimes be the case but unfortunately life is not usually so clear-cut.

The ways in which allergic reactions may contribute to asthma have been described in the section on pathophysiology (*see* page 14). The allergic trigger has been used to illustrate the various interdependent events that take place in the bronchial wall, remembering that our current knowledge is incomplete.

The magnitude of the reaction will depend upon a number of factors:

- the size of the allergen challenge;
- the extent of previous sensitization to that allergen;
- the location of primed mast cells in relation to the site of entry of the allergen;
- the precise interaction between allergen and mast cells at any given time.

The nature of the reaction – urticaria, rhinitis, conjunctivitis, asthma or anaphylaxis – will also depend upon these factors. Management would be so much easier if the allergic component of asthma involved only the early asthmatic response. What dictates whether there will be an early or a dual response? The inheritance of atopy is by an autosomal dominant gene—the difference between the early and dual responses could depend upon heterozygosity or homozygosity for atopy. Alternatively, it could depend upon a wholly different characteristic.

Why are the genes for atopy so common? It may be that other elements of the atopic state bestow advantages upon the possessors of these genes, accounting for their survival during the evolutionary process in such a high proportion of the population.

The possible role of the respiratory syncytial virus (RSV), which can cause severe bronchiolitis in infancy, in the causation of asthma in childhood is also interesting. Certainly IgE may be seen in relation to RSV particles. It has been suggested that many children who have suffered from RSV bronchiolitis subsequently develop asthma. Any interaction between the virus and the child which may lead to the development of asthma will depend upon either:

1 the RS virus preconditioning the bronchi of atopic children so that they are more likely to develop asthma subsequently; *or*
2 atopic, potentially asthmatic children being worse affected by RSV infections.

Inhaled and ingested allergens

The routes by which allergens enter the body may affect the body's response.

Inhaled allergens

The most common way for allergens to provoke asthma is via inhalation. The allergen particles have to be sufficiently small to reach and to be deposited in the small bronchi and bronchioles. The most common inhaled allergens come from the house dust mite or its faeces, pollens, fungal spores, household pets and other animals and the many specific allergens associated with occupational asthma. The house dust mite, *Dermatophagoides pteronyssimus* is a sensitizing agent for many atopic asthmatics. It lives on desquamated skin cells and its survival is encouraged by modern lifestyles, in warm, humid, well-insulated homes. Pollens and fungal spores are seasonal and their levels also depend upon the weather. Hedgerow and tree flowers pollinate in the spring and early summer, whereas grasses do so throughout the summer. Late summer and early autumn witness a surge in fungal spores. Weather is an important factor. Some fungi, for instance, release their spores in sunshine, whereas others do so specifically when it rains (either type of fungus may be found commonly on late-standing cereal crops).

Allergen avoidance may be possible, especially if an occupational allergen is involved or a pet whose role as a significant trigger has been demonstrated. Avoidance must be properly thought through and organized; the avoidance of most airborne allergens is not compatible with leading a normal life. Even the most obsessional measures do not guarantee success. For example, if a pet is implicated, then the animal in question needs to be removed from the home for 2 to 3 months, to allow the allergens from dander (dogs) or salivary proteins from preening (cats), to disappear. Reactions to individual breeds vary, so skin-tests to dogs or cats in general may be quite misleading.

Therapy to suppress the body's inappropriate responses to inhaled and other allergens is most likely to be successful. Efforts have been made in the past to 'desensitize' or 'hyposensitize' both asthmatics and hay fever sufferers with courses of injections of allergen extracts. Evidence suggested that some hay fever sufferers benefited from such courses, but the results are not reliable or predictable. Atopic individuals are likely to respond to many allergens and the natural history of the reactions depends upon the behaviour of the allergen with time and upon changes in the individual. Unfortunately, especially when the hay fever sufferer is also asthmatic, there is the small but potential risk of a fatal reaction to even a small dose of allergen. Consequently, the technique is currently little used in the United Kingdom.

Ingested allergens

The ingestion of allergens is most often associated with systemic reactions, for instance urticaria, angioneurotic oedema or even anaphylaxis. Angioneurotic oedema is similar to urticaria but occurs more extensively and more deeply within the tissues, and it can lead to obstruction of the airway at the laryngopharyngeal level.

Again, the reactions are individually specific and may occur with soft fruit, nuts, shellfish, fish, fizzy drinks, milk, beers or wines and spirits. Food and drink additives such as tartrazine have been popularly associated with such reactions, but these responses are not uncommon in the absence of additives.

Both early and late asthmatic responses may occur, or if the dose of allergen is insufficient to cause clinical asthma it may be enough to provoke bronchial hyperreactivity. In one study, Asian children were found to be more likely to suffer from bronchial hyperreactivity in response to ice, fizzy drinks, fried foods, nuts and orange squash than Caucasian children. If there is a late response or hyperreactivity, the asthma sufferer may not always associate the cause with the delayed effect.

If the food or drink can be positively identified, allergen avoidance is a sensible proposition and far more likely to meet with success than when the allergen is airborne. Occasionally, the removal of such an ingested allergen may reduce the level of bronchial hyperreactivity considerably. However, one must alert those patients or their relatives who embark upon a vain pursuit of food allergen. Such patients, intent upon a cure for their asthma, may be treated by non-medically qualified individuals. Sometimes these patients can be induced to stop their essential treatment by 'practitioners' who have little if any knowledge of the consequences of such action. Patients with chronic symptomatic conditions and a variable natural history are particularly vulnerable to these alternative practitioners who may promise a cure, thus providing another cogent reason for members of the medical and nursing professions to explain conditions such as asthma, so that patients' expectations are reasonable and they understand the role of therapy.

Exercise

Exercise-induced asthma is common and troublesome. It is a condition that has long been recognized, especially by patients. As with many aspects of asthma, the mechanisms have become less clear as our knowledge has increased. We have yet to explain the effects of air temperature and humidity and other observations on the interaction between allergen-induced and exercise-induced asthma and the effects of repeated short bursts of exercise.

A short period of exercise is usually associated with an initial rise in PEFR, then a decline which is maximal after about 5 – 7 minutes. In the majority of asthmatics, this appears to be related to the release of mast cell mediators and is accompanied by the detection of neutrophil chemotactic factor in the peripheral blood (a marker of mast cell degranulation). Part of this process of mediator release appears to depend upon cooling and drying of the bronchial mucosa, but in the majority of subjects exercise-induced asthma can also cause mediator release independently of temperature and humidity. It is possible that cooling modulates the vagal tone in the bronchi, in this case by increasing it, so that the exercise-released mediators from the smaller airways cause clinical airflow limitation with a fall in PEFR. It is well known that short bursts of activity lead to a refractory state during which further exercise fails to elicit symptoms, probably due to the depletion of mediator stores which must be replenished over the next 1 – 3 hours, before the subject is once more susceptible to exercise-induced asthma.

Thus, exercise-induced asthma can be prevented most effectively by the inhalation of sodium cromoglycate, nedocromil sodium or a $beta_2$-agonist, immediately prior to exercise. Their mode of action is related to the blocking of the degranulation of mast cells.

In summary, the mechanism of exercise-induced asthma arises predominantly from mast cell degranulation, with some influence from neural routes. Its time-course is very similar to that of the early asthmatic response of allergen-induced asthma, but exercise-induced asthma never gives rise to a picture similar to the late asthmatic response.

The general suppression of background bronchial hyperreactivity reduces the likelihood of exercise-induced asthma occurring and its severity, although it does not inhibit it. This is compatible with the concept that the higher the threshold for bronchial hyperreactivity the greater the trigger factor required to provoke clinical asthma and a fall in PEFR; conversely, the lower the threshold for bronchial hyperreactivity the smaller the trigger required.

Laughing, hyperventilation and cold air

Laughing, coughing and hyperventilation all operate through airway cooling, i.e. the inhalation of cold air, which may itself trigger clinical asthma in the absence of exercise. For symptoms to be induced, a certain level of background hyperreactivity must also be present. These problems may be prevented by suppression of bronchial hyperreactivity or pre-treatment (*see* page 23).

Emotion

Emotion or psychological factors may trigger asthma, but by more than one mechanism. Clearly, it is common for someone who is upset to hyperventilate and this is a powerful asthma trigger. Even in the absence of hyperventilation, some asthmatics may become symptomatic, probably through the action of the vagus in increasing smooth muscle tone in the bronchi. This latter mechanism can be blocked by using ipratropium, an inhaled anticholinergic agent.

Non-specific irritants

Into this category fall agents to which the asthmatic subject is not allergic but whose presence as an irritant is sufficient to provoke coughing and wheezing. For example, non-specific dusts, powders, fumes and smoke.

Cigarette or tobacco smoke might be a non-specific irritant in that it will cause bronchial hyperreactivity, most noticeably in those who are non-smokers but who suffer immediate or delayed effects upon entering a smoky environment. Most cigarette-smoking asthmatics who stop smoking notice a marked and progressive improvement in their symptoms, occasionally being able to discontinue therapy which was necessary to counter the effects of tobacco smoke. However, there is a very small group of asthmatics who stop smoking whose symptoms initially become worse before they improve over the longer term. This may be due to the loss of the pharmacological effect of a component of tobacco smoke (perhaps that of the nicotine).

Cigarette smoking appears to increase mucosal permeability to inhaled haptens, i.e. substances that become antigens (allergens) when they associate with body proteins. In one study, twice as many smoking atopic subjects developed specific IgE when compared with a group of non-smoking atopic subjects.

Aspirin and non-steroidal anti-inflammatory drugs

The role of aspirin and non-steroidal anti-inflammatory drugs (NSAIDs) in asthma is interesting. There is evidence that NSAIDs will suppress part of the late asthmatic response to allergen challenge, which is compatible with their known action in inhibiting the cyclo-oxygenase and lipoxygenase pathways.

However, some late-onset asthmatics are sensitive to aspirin and other NSAIDs. Their asthma may be catastrophically triggered, the results of which may occasionally be fatal. This may be due to drugs' effects upon the cyclo-oxygenase and lipoxygenase pathways, thereby upsetting the balance between the products of the two. Patients who are known to be sensitive to aspirin should be warned not to purchase over-the-counter NSAIDs such as ibuprofen, which is now available as a general-purpose analgesic.

Beta-blocking drugs

As mentioned elsewhere (*see* page 4), beta-blocking drugs may precipitate asthma. This may occur when late-onset asthma begins *de novo* in a patient who has been receiving a beta-blocker for many years, or it may happen when a beta-blocker is inadvertently prescribed for a known asthmatic patient. The effects may range from mild exercise symptoms, through nocturnal symptoms, to death from severe asthma.

The effects are likely to be worse with non-selective beta-blockers, but even those with relative $beta_1$-blocking specificity may cause broncho-constriction in those whose bronchial airflow is sensitively balanced. Alternative therapy should be considered because it is not good management practice to provide additional therapy to overcome iatrogenic problems, unless it is unavoidable.

Beta-blockers should be avoided in asthmatic subjects. This applies to those agents used in the treatment of angina and hypertension, and also the ophthalmic preparations used to treat glaucoma, which are absorbed systemically.

Gastro-oesophageal reflux

It has been recognized for some years that nocturnal acid reflux could aggravate asthma and increase bronchial hyperreactivity. Sometimes, the reflux is symptomatic. Although the relationship is not straightforward, it would seem sensible to take simple measures to reduce reflux and aspiration.

1 Elevate the head of the bed.
2 Avoid late meals and late alcoholic drinks.
3 Lose weight if obesity contributes to the problem.
4 Use anti-refluxing agents such as alginate/antacid mixtures, or make a trial of H_2-receptor antagonists, such as ranitidine (cimetidine may interact with theophyllines).

Menstrual factors

Some women notice a marked deterioration in their asthma in the luteal phase of the menstrual cycle or at the start of menstruation. There is disagreement over whether hormonal or anti-hormonal therapy has a beneficial effect upon such asthma. I think that each patient should be individually assessed and therapy, such as progesterone or danazol, tried if deemed appropriate.

It is not uncommon for the severity of asthma to change during pregnancy. For some women their asthma will become less of a problem, in others it will become worse. It should be stressed to mothers-to-be that the judicious use of prophylactic therapy, when appropriate, may be beneficial to both mother and baby.

3 Clinical Recognition

Breathlessness – Wheeze – Cough – Nocturnal cough – 'Wheezy bronchitis' – Changes with age – Late onset asthma – Differential diagnosis – Other conditions can co-exist – Beware hyperventilation

Symptoms

The symptoms of asthma are not constantly present. In particular, they may not be present at the time that the asthma sufferer consults a doctor. In the past and perhaps even today, this has led to the non-diagnosis of asthma. It is imperative to take a good history and not to expect symptoms and signs on demand. Symptoms may be minimal at rest during the daytime, but severe during the night or upon exertion.

The principal symptoms of asthma are:

1 breathlessness or dyspnoea;
2 wheeze;
3 cough.

These symptoms do not necessarily occur simultaneously and *it is essential that the diagnosis of asthma is not dismissed in the absence of a wheeze.*

Dyspnoea is a disturbance of breathing when, in order to maintain a given level of ventilation, a disproportionate effort must be applied. Naturally, this becomes exaggerated during the increased respiratory demands of exercise.

The *wheeze* is caused by turbulence in the air currents within the bronchi. Turbulence depends upon the reduction in airway calibre, which occurs in asthma, and the velocity of the airflow. Thus, the wheeze may be masked by a patient who breathes quietly deliberately or because the asthma is so severe that there is insufficient airflow to create turbulence—the 'silent chest' of very severe asthma. Paradoxically, the noisiest wheeze may be associated with the least objective evidence of airflow limitation.

The *cough* may be dry, due to the stimulation of irritant receptors in the larger bronchi, or it may be productive. Mucus production is a common accompaniment to the inflammatory element of asthma. Simple mucus may be clear and mucoid, or it may be discoloured, thicker and very viscid as a result of cellular infiltration. The colour of the sputum is not a reliable guide to the presence of infection.

Age patterns

Infancy and early childhood

The commonest problems in infancy and early childhood are nocturnal cough and recurrent attacks of wheezing associated with viral respiratory tract infections.

It is often stated that it is impossible to diagnose asthma in infancy. However, there is a group of children whose nights will be regularly broken by coughing, the child often waking up breathless and wheezy with a lot of mucus; during the day, there is little or no problem. These symptoms occur in the absence of a respiratory tract infection.

Recurrent episodes of wheezing, with infection, have long been known as 'wheezy bronchitis'. These episodes start at the same time as a 'cold' with a cough, which is often dry but soon becomes 'finely moist' with a tight sound. This progresses to considerable wheezing and distress, with marked restlessness and an inability to settle, often with much mucus production. The mucus appears watery and frothy. The dyspnoea and bronchorrhoea lead to aerophagy with subsequent gastric distension and further breathlessness, but vomiting, which frequently occurs, affords temporary partial relief. These episodes usually last for several days, the first and second nights being the worst.

Coughing and breathlessness on exertion in the absence of a respiratory tract infection do occur, but their appearance depends as much on the child's general development and level of activity as on the natural history of asthma.

Symptoms may be very mild and may cause little if any trouble to the child, but they can be very upsetting for the parents who are considering the wider implications. However, symptoms can be severe and may lead to hospital admission. There is a striking preponderance of asthma in boys at this age.

Later childhood

With increased activities, children become more aware of the physical limitations from their exercise-induced symptoms, which in the absence of effective therapy may prevent them from taking part in games and sports. Problems from nocturnal disturbance and respiratory infections will continue if no effective treatment is offered. The number of girls affected begins to increase at this age. Some children will experience seasonal exacerbations associated with allergic reactions to airborne allergens, such as pollens and fungal spores.

Adolescence

In common with many conditions, asthma often changes at or around puberty. Some patients will present for the first time; many will experience fewer symptoms or even become free of them. This applies particularly to those who have been affected primarily by viral respiratory tract infections.

Although it is tempting to suggest that a child will 'grow out of' his or her asthma, no-one can predict with any degree of certainty that a child will lose his or her symptoms, even if there is a general improvement throughout adolescence. Those who have had prominent atopic symptoms are least likely to become symptom-free. Patients who are led to believe that their symptoms will disappear are likely to lose faith in their medical attendants if the symptoms remain.

Adulthood

Early adult life may herald the return of symptoms in some asthmatics, often related to exercise or in association with seasonal factors such as inhaled allergens, the third decade seeing the highest level of IgE-associated problems. Some adult asthmatics may have been symptomatic from childhood, but such symptoms will usually be controllable with treatment.

The middle-aged and elderly may develop late-onset asthma *de novo*. Not uncommonly, it follows a severe episode of 'bronchitis' or pulmonary infection from which there may be a slow but full recovery, only for symptoms to return, with breathlessness, wheezing and nocturnal symptoms (which may be the most severe feature). Frequently, patients suffer intolerable symptoms before they report them, most commonly because they assume it is a part of the ageing process or their 'due' as a result of having smoked. In this age group, the sex ratio of sufferers approaches a balance as there are relatively more female sufferers among the late presenters.

Many adults who develop asthma have been diagnosed as having 'bronchitis' even if they have never smoked and neither lived nor worked in an injurious environment. This misdiagnosis leads to a negative therapeutic approach and a diagnosis of asthma should always be borne in mind. Tobacco-smokers can and do develop asthma which must be recognized for what it is.

Differential diagnosis

The importance of discussing differential diagnosis is twofold:

1 to consider the other diagnostic possibilities when a patient presents with breathlessness, cough and wheeze;
2 to remember that asthma sufferers receiving regular care and follow-up are not immune to the conditions affecting any other members of the community. Thus, a worsening of the symptoms may not be due solely to the asthma.

The differential diagnosis changes with the patient's age and circumstances, but treatment must be tailored to meet the patient's condition. Diagnoses will be considered according to what may occur at (a) any age, (b) in childhood or (c) in adult life.

Any age

1 Acute bronchitis or bronchiolitis.
2 Bronchial obstruction.
3 Bronchiectasis.
4 Hyperventilation.

Acute bronchitis or bronchiolitis

Acute bronchitis in response to a viral infection does not usually affect the same patient more than once in a few years unless a patient is predisposed to over-react to these infections, as in asthma. In both children and adults, it is important to await the unfolding of the natural history of the condition. Anyone can be wise in retrospect and so the first episode of bronchitis or bronchiolitis may prove to be the herald for asthma, but this cannot be assumed at the start. Thus, keep an open mind in the presence of wheeze, breathlessness, cough, debility, fever and sputum production.

Bronchiolitis in infancy is particularly difficult as it is indistinguishable from later episodes of asthma. Bronchiolitis is most often associated with RSV infections and can be responsible for a distressing illness. A large proportion of children affected can be subject to repeated episodes of wheezing caused by respiratory tract viruses and bronchial hyperreactivity for many years. It is not known whether RSV causes these problems in normal babies and children, or whether atopic children are more susceptible to the effects of RSV and its sequelae.

Bronchial obstruction

Although the causes of bronchial obstruction may be different in adults and children, in both it may present dramatically and acutely with a cough and noisy breathing, the timing of which depends upon the site of obstruction and other considerations. A confounding factor may be its occurrence in an asthmatic (not unlikely when one considers the prevalence of asthma).

In adults, the most likely causes are neoplasms, benign or malignant, which may lie within the bronchus or cause pressure from outside the bronchus, such as that from an enlarged lymph node or a tumour. Sometimes there may be a preceding history of a cough or even haemoptysis, and a solitary wheeze may be heard over the narrowed bronchus before it is totally obstructed. There may be other enlarged glands, such as in the neck, or associated phenomena such as 'finger-clubbing'. The possibility of tracheal compression from a goitre, possibly retrosternal, should be borne in mind.

In children the commonest cause of bronchial obstruction is an inhaled foreign body such as a bead, a piece of a plastic toy or a peanut. Sometimes the consequences develop rapidly but it can be weeks or years before the foreign body causes symptoms. Usually there will be respiratory distress and the time available for treatment is governed by the site at which the object becomes lodged. If it causes total obstruction of the bronchus, there will be progressive absorption of air from that lobe or segment, with a shift of the heart and mediastinum to that side. If there is a valve-effect, then air can enter but not leave that lobe which leads to lobar emphysema with pressure on the other lung and a shift of the mediastinum away from the affected side.

Urgent admission for X-ray and bronchoscopy is necessary, bearing in mind that it is exceptional for the foreign body to be radio-opaque.

Bronchiectasis

Although more common in adults, bronchiectasis does occur in children. Its name derives from the dilatation of bronchi, due to damage to their walls, either locally or throughout wide areas of the lungs. This dilatation, together with the replacement of the normal ciliated type of epithelium with a squamous type in the dilated areas, leads to the pooling of bronchial secretions in the dependent zones of the lungs. There may be a productive cough, with sputum which can be clear to deeply discoloured, yellow or green, and perhaps episodic segmental infection and pleurisy. The cough is affected by position because retained secretions drain to larger tubes to be expectorated. Sometimes there may be an association with asthma, in which bronchiectasis heightens the bronchial hyperreactivity and the inflammatory processes of the asthma thereby increasing the mucus load of the bronchiectasis. Each problem warrants specific treatment; bronchiectasis requires postural drainage, 'huffing' and antibiotics. Sometimes a local patch of bronchiectasis may simply alter the normal respiratory dynamics and lead to hyperventilation.

Bronchiectasis may be secondary to severe pertussis, pneumonia, measles or pulmonary tuberculosis, or it may be associated with immunodeficiency disorders or immotile cilia syndromes. In the immotile cilia syndromes, there are likely to be recurrent sinus problems, adding to the pulmonary disorders from nocturnal overspill and post-nasal drip. Immunodeficiency leads to a heavier bacterial load and local infection with ensuing damage, whereas immotile cilia allow pooling of secretions (the bronchial mucus collects rather than being propelled towards the pharynx). Pooling may result in bacterial overgrowth in normally sterile areas of the respiratory tract.

Bronchiectasis may mimic asthma by causing a nocturnal cough, which is usually posture-induced, and by being associated with wheezing caused by bacterial bronchitis. The latter may respond quickly to antibiotics which would not be the case with asthma.

Hyperventilation

Hyperventilation can lead to diagnostic confusion: it can occur in isolation or it may represent only one symptom of a respiratory disorder. It should not be viewed as an hysterical phenomenon. Fear will increase the level of hyperventilation, which can be very noisy thereby leading to misdiagnosis as asthma.

Hyperventilation can occur at any age. It must be distinguished from:

1 true dyspnoea;
2 appropriate tachypnoea, for example, in response to exercise;
3 secondary tachypnoea, as in response to a metabolic acidosis.

Hyperventilation is a breathing pattern that is too rapid and too deep for the demands of the moment. It does not increase oxygenation of the blood, but leads to hypocapnia (reduced pCO_2) and its subsequent effects. Hyperventilation may be triggered by pain, fear, anxiety, unrecognized pulmonary problems or true dyspnoea, such as the onset of asthma with increased airflow resistance. Diagnostic confusion may arise because hyperventilation may provoke asthma or make it worse, thereby setting up a vicious circle.

It may require a great deal of skill to disentangle the condition of hyperventilation from other problems. It is important to explain its mechanism and effects to the patient so that they recognize it and are not afraid of its effects. Useful tests are tidal breathing records, estimation of arterial blood gases and PEFR measurements at the time of symptoms, ensuring that the expiratory effort is genuinely maximal.

Low-grade hyperventilation may lead to tiredness, dizziness, tinnitus and blurred vision. If more acute, it may cause tingling (paraesthesiae) in the hands, feet and face, particularly around the mouth, with muscle stiffness and a sense of losing control. Occasionally, it leads to de-personalization, detachment, unconsciousness and fits, all the result of hypocapnia and alkalosis. Being able to understand the problem is sufficient treatment for many patients, but to allay the effects of hyperventilation the patient should re-breathe expired air from a paper bag. This manoeuvre allows the carbon dioxide to re-equilibrate.

Caution should be practised when treating asthmatics who hyperventilate. Physiotherapists may have a useful role in instructing patients how not to hyperventilate when their asthma increases in severity because it can lead to a feeling of losing control and worsens the patient's condition.

Childhood

1 Croup/inspiratory stridor.
2 Cystic fibrosis.

Croup/inspiratory stridor

The characteristic sign of croup is a noisy inspiration through a narrowed laryngopharynx followed by a cough similar to the bark of a sealion.

The sudden onset of a first attack of croup is most alarming for both the child and his or her parents. This fear can be infectious and aggravates the symptoms as respiratory demands increase. The commonest causes of croup are respiratory viruses that cause laryngitis, which often affect the same child repeatedly. The outcome is usually benign, but if the obstruction is serious there will be intercostal recession during quiet inspiration.

A serious potentially fatal cause of croup is epiglottitis due to *Haemophilus influenzae*, which demands urgent admission, intubation or tracheotomy, and parenteral antibiotics.

Cystic fibrosis

Cystic fibrosis is the most common recessively inherited disorder in the United Kingdom. It is chronic, with recurrent chest infections, failure to thrive and evidence of malabsorption. There is one case in approximately 2000 live births in the United Kingdom.

The chest infections will usually be severe and protracted, with fever, cough and wheeze and lead to lung damage. Radiological changes will be found on chest X-ray. In children a sweat test reveals high levels of sodium (>70 mmol/litre). Abnormalities of mucus secretion result in a susceptibility to pulmonary infections. Moreover, the child is usually not fit and well in other respects. The outlook has improved immeasurably over the past twenty years.

Nowadays children survive into their late teens and adult life, but at a physical price—regular ingestion of antibiotics to prevent colonization by pathogens and daily physiotherapy at school and at home to drain secretions. Some patients may be suitable for heart – lung transplantation. In future, antenatal screening and genetic engineering may reduce the incidence of this condition. Some cystic fibrosis sufferers may reach adult life before the diagnosis is made, having had repeated chest infections treated unsuccessfully in the past.

Adulthood

The picture seen in respiratory disease in adult life is complicated by the problems of ageing, the effects of home and occupational environments and the effects of smoking.

1 Pulmonary oedema.
2 Irreversible airflow limitation.
3 Parenchymal lung disease.

Pulmonary oedema

Although pulmonary oedema may occur after exposure to some poisonous fumes, it is seen most commonly in the presence of left ventricular failure or mitral stenosis.

The symptoms may mimic asthma and it may be impossible to distinguish between pulmonary oedema and acute severe nocturnal asthma when called in the early hours of the morning to a new patient without the performance of further tests, which requires hospital admission. Often there will be a history of preceding exercise dyspnoea. In pulmonary oedema, the patient is woken in the early hours (usually slightly earlier than with asthma), severely breathless, and is unable to lie down (orthopnoea); he or she is wheezing and coughing, often producing white or, less commonly, pink froth and may be cyanosed. Presentation in the daytime is generally less severe and more subtle.

It is essential to monitor the heart, blood pressure, heart rate and rhythm, because hypertension and dysrhythmias are common causes of left ventricular failure. An electrocardiogram (ECG) and a chest X-ray will be helpful but the latter may not be available instantly. In addition to ischaemic heart disease and valvular heart disease, severe anaemia can cause left ventricular failure, when the heart can no longer compensate. In a younger patient, severe anaemia may cause breathlessness and tachycardia disproportionate to the exertion.

Irreversible airflow limitation

Irreversible airflow limitation is usually associated with the 'chronic bronchitis' and 'emphysema' secondary to years of smoking. Considerable damage to the lungs will have occurred before presentation. However, it must not be forgotten that asthma itself, if left untreated for years, can lead to irreversible damage to the bronchial tree (although this condition will have been symptomatic throughout the subject's life).

There will be various combinations of the following symptoms: breathlessness (the most prominent), cough, wheeze, sputum and possibly cyanosis. It is important to prohibit smoking if the patient has any genuine desire to improve. Smoking will add to the progressive lung damage, while carbon monoxide competes with oxygen for transport in the blood which adds to the level of hypoxaemia, thereby reducing exercise capacity and increasing the likelihood of pulmonary hypertension developing, with consequent right heart failure.

Some young patients may suffer an accelerated form of predominantly basal emphysema related to $alpha_1$ antitrypsin deficiency. Although the level of $alpha_1$ antitrypsin can be measured in the blood by the GP, full assessment should be performed under the instruction of a respiratory physician.

Before it can be assumed that irreversible disease is present, it is imperative that the full battery of reversibility tests is performed, not just with nebulized bronchodilators but with the administration for 2 – 3 weeks of adequate amounts of systemic corticosteroids (*see* page 81). It is not sufficient to rely on subjective improvements, particularly as no patient will be grateful if left on high doses of corticosteroids and then develops long-term side effects such as collapsed vertebrae, from ineffective therapy. However, some asthmatic patients with irreversibility may be helped by prophylactic therapy to prevent further deterioration.

Parenchymal lung disease

Disorders of entirely different aetiology may present in similar ways, principally because the lungs display a limited repertoire of symptom complexes. Their onset may be insidious or acute, sometimes associated with a cough and wheeze, but certainly with breathlessness. Sometimes the physical signs may be unimpressive, possibly an occasional wheeze or, in fibrosing alveolitis, fine inspiratory crackles can be heard particularly at the bases of the lungs. Radiological signs may be characteristic, and respiratory function tests will show evidence of restricted volume and diminished gas transfer (an indirect measure of oxygen uptake).

These diseases may be associated with multisystem problems or may occur only in the lungs, for example:

1 alveolitis—allergic or cryptogenic, fibrosing;
2 polyarteritis nodosa;

3 sarcoidosis;
4 systemic sclerosis (scleroderma).

These conditions are not common in comparison with asthma and although the diagnoses may be made by GPs it is important that they are managed by respiratory physicians.

4 Complications of Asthma

Pneumothorax – Mediastinal emphysema – Atelectasis – Allergic bronchopulmonary aspergillosis – Chest deformity – Growth suppression – Delayed puberty and growth spurt – Irreversibility

In general, the complications of asthma are more likely to occur in those patients who have the most severe asthma. Some complications will be the result of severe acute asthma, whereas others will reflect the chronic nature of much asthma.

Acute complications

1 Pneumothorax.
2 Mediastinal emphysema.
3 Atelectasis secondary to mucus-plugging.
4 Allergic bronchopulmonary aspergillosis.

Pneumothorax

During an attack of severe acute asthma, with marked hyperinflation, a subpleural alveolus may burst into the pleural cavity (Fig. 4.1, *see* overleaf). This allows air to enter the pleural cavity and can have two possible results.

1 Partial collapse of that lung due to the loss of the relatively negative pressure in the pleural cavity, but stabilization occurs with equilibration.
2 A tension pneumothorax, in which a valve-effect allows air to enter the pleural cavity, but no air can escape to equilibrate, thereby building up a positive pressure in that pleural cavity sufficient to compress the adjacent lung and shift the mediastinum to the opposite side. The outcome is potentially fatal.

The immediate effect of a pneumothorax is an acute increase in dyspnoea which is both reflex and due to reduced oxygenation of the blood. The

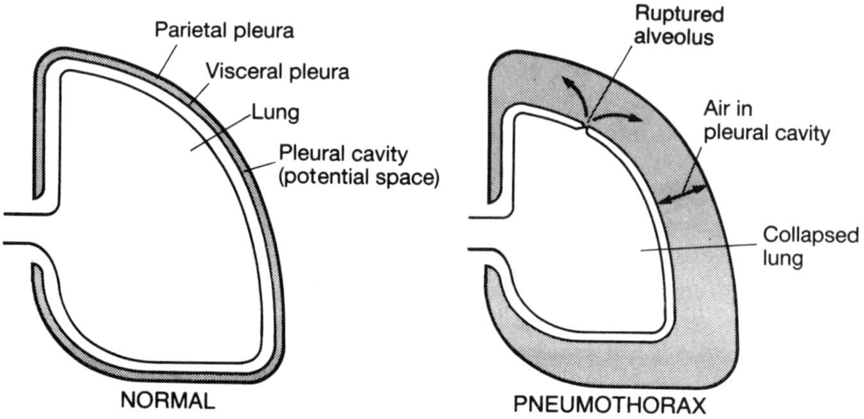

Figure 4.1 Diagram to illustrate a pneumothorax.

physical signs are of diminished chest movement on the affected side with reduced breath sounds and vocal fremitus and hyperresonance on percussion. A tension pneumothorax will shift the trachea and apex beat to the opposite side and may need urgent release via a needle if there is any delay before admission to hospital.

A chest X-ray will confirm the diagnosis.

Mediastinal emphysema

Sometimes an alveolus may rupture but the pleura remains intact so that the escaping air tracks along the bronchi, enters the mediastinum and then spreads in all directions (Fig. 4.2), particularly rising to throat and face (Fig. 8.2, *see* page 106). The palpable crackle or crepitus of surgical emphysema can be detected. The air will reabsorb spontaneously but the process can be hastened by breathing oxygen-enriched air.

Atelectasis secondary to mucus-plugging

During a protracted exacerbation of asthma that includes increased mucus production, it is not uncommon for a plug of mucus to occlude a bronchial division, especially in children. This leads to atelectasis, with the collapse of the segment or lobe served by that bronchus, as the air is progressively absorbed. Atelectasis will resolve with intensive treatment of the asthma and physiotherapy.

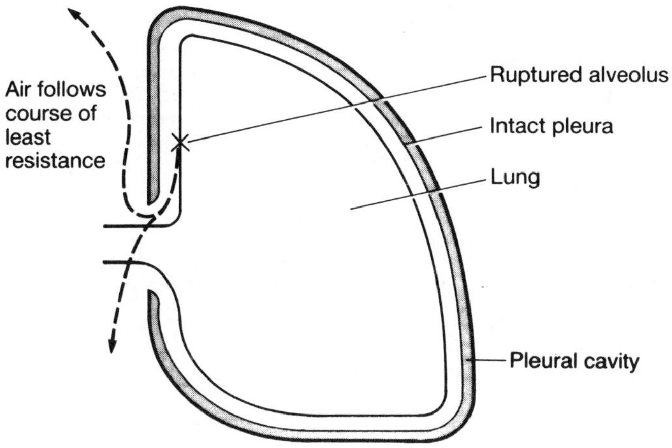

Figure 4.2 Diagram to illustrate mediastinal emphysema.

Allergic bronchopulmonary aspergillosis

Allergic bronchopulmonary aspergillosis is an intense allergic response of sensitive asthmatic lungs to the presence of the ubiquitous fungus *Aspergillus*. The fungal hyphae adhere to the bronchial epithelium and provoke a reaction, with eosinophilic infiltration and damage to the bronchial wall. Plugging of bronchi with possible collapse and consolidation will be visible radiologically. The sputum characteristically contains odd brownish plugs.

If left untreated (systemic corticosteroids suppress the reaction to *Aspergillus*), considerable damage to bronchi occurs, with dilatation and bronchiectasis. Blood may show an eosinophilia, very high levels of IgE and precipitins to *Aspergillus*.

Chronic complications

Although the first two chronic complications of asthma occur only in childhood asthma, the third may occur at any age. All are a reflection of severity.

1 Chest deformity.
2 Disturbances of growth and development.
3 Progression to irreversibility.

Chest deformity

Persistent untreated asthma in childhood may lead to a chest wall deformity. The ribs are malleable and the muscles of respiration pull in various directions, so the shape of the chest is a compromise between the barrel-shaped hyperinflated upper chest and the drawing in of the lower ribs, with an exaggerated Harrison's sulcus, secondary to the pull of the diaphragm.

Disturbances of growth and development

Provided that an adequate number of readings is taken, a chart plotting a child's growth is a sensitive index of his or her well-being. Uncontrolled asthma is associated with suppressed growth. Growth hormone is normally released in bursts during vigorous exercise and REM sleep, both of which are affected by uncontrolled chronic asthma.

The prolonged use of systemic corticosteroids is also associated with growth suppression. With the advent of effective prophylactic therapy, the use of protracted courses of systemic corticosteroids in childhood asthma is now very rare. However, caution should be exercised. Although the inhaled corticosteroid, beclomethasone, does not appear to affect growth adversely in dosages up to 600 μg/day, when increasing the dosage weigh up all the considerations first, especially whether the drug is being appropriately used and in a safe dosage. The objective should be minimum therapy for the desired effect.

An interesting phenomenon is that of delayed puberty in relation to atopy, even if the atopic problems are mild. The appearance of secondary sexual characteristics and the adolescent growth spurt are delayed, and growth continues at its childhood level. When puberty and the growth spurt do occur, the ultimate height achieved is at least that predicted from earlier growth performance and it can be above average.

Progression to irreversibility

It has long been known that smoking leads to permanent lung damage, by stimulating mucous gland hyperplasia and encouraging the destructive effects of proteolytic enzymes released by inflammatory cells in the lungs. However, a chronic asthmatic process can lead to irreversible airflow limitation that has no significant response to either bronchodilators or corticosteroids. Consider the inflammatory reaction in asthma: usually mediators are considered in terms of bronchoconstriction, capillary permeability and mucus production but the destructive potential of the inflammatory cells must be borne in mind. Some of the mediators are cytotoxic, but several proteolytic and other enzymes are present in the granules of granulocytes. There is smooth muscle hypertrophy, but beneath the epithelium even the basement membrane is thickened by the deposition of collagen by fibroblasts. Just as in other inflammatory reactions which are unchecked, the end result is akin to scarring.

5 Tests of Lung Function

Measurements mandatory – Tests subject to errors – PEFR – Spirometry – FEV_1 – FVC – Consistent technique – Home monitoring of PEFR – Equipment – Exercise test – Reversibility tests – Avoid provocation tests

Who would treat hypertension without regular measurement of blood pressure? Who indeed would manage diabetes mellitus without some reflection of the metabolic state? In the past diabetic patients relied upon their own measurements of urinary glucose concentration, but now insulin-dependent diabetics monitor their blood glucose to assist in their own fine-tuning of insulin dosage. Their medical attendants make judgements using both the patient's results and estimations of glycosylated haemoglobin. Why then are there still doctors whose diagnosis and treatment of asthma rests solely upon the presence of a wheeze on auscultation of the chest, with the patient's symptoms sometimes taken into account?

Lung function

Asthma is a disorder of function. Oversensitive pulmonary airways become narrowed, thereby increasing the resistance to flow and restricting airflow both into and especially out of the lungs. The patient's account of his or her symptoms and their replies to direct questions will elucidate when symptoms occur, perhaps why they occur and also the extent to which they affect the patient's lifestyle. The history will be sufficient to make a diagnosis of asthma in the majority of cases. However, the patient's concept of his or her symptoms and auscultation of the chest are not reliable indicators of the severity of asthma. It is well recognized that a silent chest may be an indication of very severe asthma and not simply of the absence of asthma. A subjective assessment of symptoms will not establish a stable baseline. After a period of effective therapy, symptoms of asthma that were quite acceptable to the patient three months before will be quite intolerable, as expectations will have rightly changed.

Thus, there must be a reproducible objective measure of pulmonary function, with particular reference to the airways. Whatever parameters are selected, to make the results reproducible within the individual and therefore meaningful, it should be remembered that these measurements depend on a number of non-clinical factors:

- age;
- sex;
- height;
- build;
- posture;
- patient effort.

Age, sex, height and build are unalterable. However, the observer must insist that the patient's posture is consistent. Unless there are overriding considerations, the patient should be standing when the tests are carried out. Anyone with significant hyperinflation or an obese abdomen will exhibit restricted movement of the diaphragm when seated, which will adversely affect the results obtained.

However, the most common source of fallibility in lung function testing is the variability of patient effort. It is essential that the subject understands the aims of the test and has been well instructed in what is required, preferably assisted by a demonstration by the observer. Apart from faulty technique and the failure to pay attention to detail, some subjects, especially those who hyperventilate, find it difficult to produce consistent results. On occasions, paradoxical results may be obtained that can be quite misleading.

Whatever tests are used, there are wide limits of normality—quoted figures are always mean values and there is variation among sources, depending on the authors, the year and the population studied. 'Ethnic corrections' can be applied, but they should not be used to justify the acceptance of mediocre results in a patient who is capable of better results. Although mean values are useful, within-patient results are the most instructive in that they allow comparisons to be made between the patient's present and past performances.

The parameters of lung function chosen to aid in the diagnosis and monitoring of asthma must be easy to apply in everyday clinical practice. The most convenient tests are those taken during forced expiration, such as the peak expiratory flow rate (PEFR), the forced expiratory volume in one second (FEV_1) and the forced vital capacity (FVC). On theoretical grounds, there are other tests which may appear to be more appropriate measures of the function of airways of different calibre, but none of them are as convenient or reproducible as those mentioned above. Occasionally, examination of the flow–volume loop may help to distinguish asthma from other causes of airflow limitation. Modern technology has provided us with equipment that ranges from the cheap and simple to the expensive and complex; much valuable information comes from devices costing under £20, while equipment costing almost £2000 will provide more information than is necessary. The clinician must not be distracted by digital displays and print-outs, when the pitfalls depend upon human fallibility.

Peak expiratory flow rate

The simplest measurement that can be applied to subjects with asthma is that of the PEFR, i.e. the maximum rate of expiration, maintained for 10 milliseconds, that occurs within about the first second of forced expiration (Fig. 5.1a). This obviates the need to continue to the end of expiration. PEFR is measured most easily with a Wright peak flow meter or a mini-Wright peak flow meter, calibrated for either low or normal ranges (Fig. 5.1).

Most of the resistance to airflow in a normal subject is found in the larger airways, where flow is also more turbulent. As the bronchial tree divides, the cross-sectional area of the bronchi and bronchioles increases greatly in comparison with the trachea and main bronchi; thus, the peripheral resistance to flow is very low. In the presence of the narrowing of airways of whatever calibre, there is a slowing of bronchial airflow and during forced expiration some of the smaller airways will close, trapping air peripherally. In asthma therefore, the narrowing of small airways will contribute to the lowering of the PEFR.

It is essential to pay attention to technique—PEFR is a measurement taken during the effort-dependent phase of forced expiration.

Method

1 Ensure that the patient is standing.
2 Check that the needle or pointer of the peak flow meter is on zero.
3 Instruct the patient to take as deep a breath as is possible.
4 Put the mouthpiece between the lips, which must be sealed tightly around it.
5 Holding the meter horizontally, the patient should blow out as hard as is possible.
6 Read the position of the needle or pointer.
7 Take the best of three readings.

Some subjects will prepare themselves for the test by taking repeated deep breaths, a manoeuvre akin to hyperventilation which will often aggravate the situation if they are unstable asthmatics—by the time a result is obtained, the PEFR may be lower than when the test procedure was commenced.

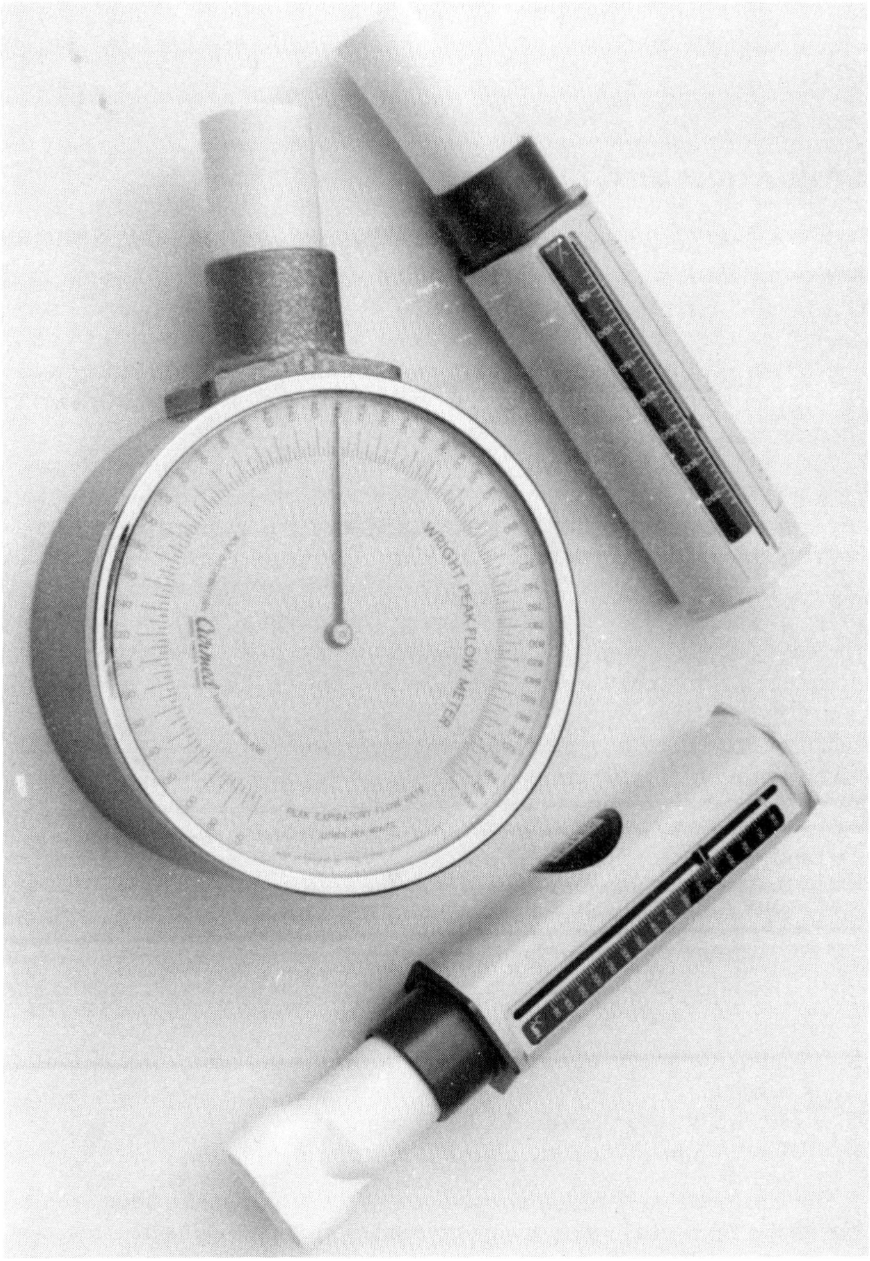

Figure 5.1 Peak flow meters.

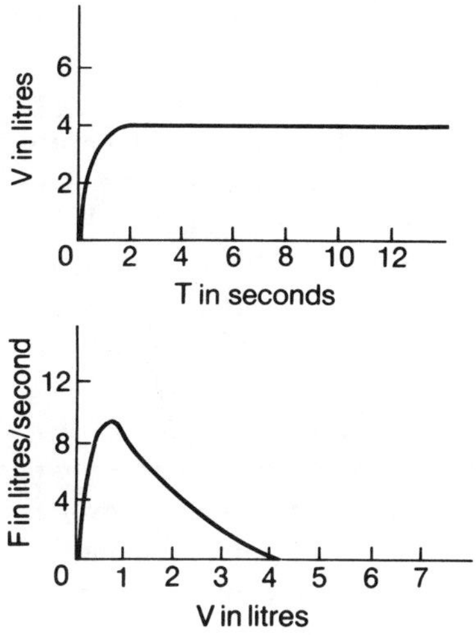

Figure 5.1a Normal spirogram above a normal expiratory flow-volume curve.

Sources of error

1 Failure of patient to take a full breath.
2 Failure to seal the lips.
3 Patient's concern over the mouthpiece, loose false teeth, etc.
4 Escape of air down the patient's nose.
5 Faulty technique on the part of the patient:
   i poor effort;
   ii protracted, low-force blow;
   iii 'cheek-blowing' or 'spitting air' which may artificially raise the poor results of those with extensive pulmonary disease.
6 Rarely, the piston may stick and yield no result, or it may suddenly release and shoot past the true value with a dull crack.

The advantages of the peak flow meter are that it is cheap, compact and ideally suited to monitoring a dynamic disorder such as asthma. It is of more value to match symptoms to the PEFR than to perform spirometry on a solitary occasion when symptoms may be absent.

Home monitoring of the peak expiratory flow rate

The asthmatic patient does not always show evidence of airflow limitation; any recording of lung function is instantaneous. Although the interpretation of a result is important, it must be viewed within the context of the patient's natural history. If a test in the surgery is normal in the absence of symptoms, the diagnosis cannot be rejected, but rather evidence of variability in the PEFR should be sought. Variation in the PEFR of 15% is considered to be significant.

Home monitoring of the PEFR can be carried out easily and it is especially valuable if the results are displayed graphically (Fig. 5.2, *see* next page). The results may be used to aid diagnosis or to monitor specific changes after the diagnosis has been accepted. The best times at which to take readings are on rising, in the afternoon, before retiring to bed and during any nocturnal disturbance—the 'morning dip'. If the patient is using an inhaled bronchodilator, it is useful to take measurements before and after inhalation.

Non-asthmatics also show some variation in PEFR, the lowest values being recorded in the early hours of the morning and on getting out of bed. Values then rise and remain at a steady level throughout the day. The amount of variation is small, usually around 5%. In the presence of bronchial hyperreactivity, the 'morning dip' is exaggerated and the PEFR may fall catastrophically, perhaps by 75% not a mere 15%. It is not known why the 'morning dip' occurs and it is unlikely that the explanation is simple. There is circumstantial evidence that the 'morning dip' coincides with low levels of circulating catecholamines and of endogenous corticosteroids, as well as a peak in serum histamine levels. There have been reports of beneficial effects from the use if ipratropium, thereby indicating that there may be a vagal component in some patients.

After effective control of their asthma, most patients, even those who had accepted a very restricted lifestyle, will regain some insight into how their lungs 'feel', especially if they can match their own sensations with PEFR readings—what I call 'resetting the bronchostats'. Those patients who are more obsessional will feel more secure if they carry out regular PEFR measurements and chart them, but this is not necessary for most asthmatics. Random tests, especially if performed in the morning or after exercise, are usually sufficient, unless the patient is aware of a change, such as the occurrence of a cough, breathlessness, a tight chest on exertion or waking in the night. If there is a deviation from normal, regular recordings can be resumed to monitor the patient's condition. PEFR recordings have no intrinsic value and they should be viewed as a form of information which may or may not warrant subsequent action. As will be discussed later in the section on management (*see* p. 99), the aim of therapy and monitoring is to ensure optimum levels of function; to achieve this, active adjustment of therapy will be necessary. All too often, declining lung function is observed without active intervention. Any decline in function should be arrested as soon as possible.

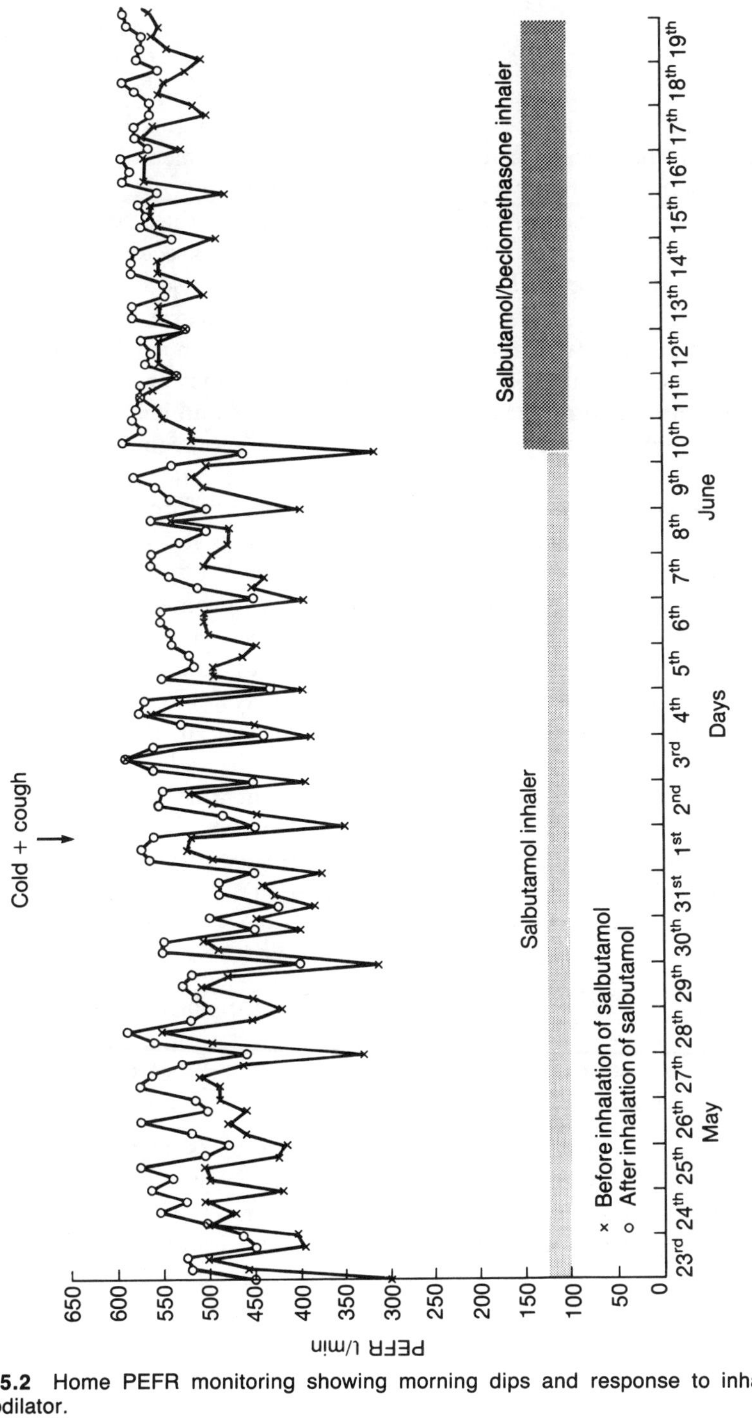

Figure 5.2 Home PEFR monitoring showing morning dips and response to inhaled bronchodilator.

Spirometry

Spirometry relies upon volume measurement during expiration. It is most commonly performed using a dry-bellows device such as the Vitalograph which produces a tracing of volume against time (Fig. 5.3a, *see* next page). The passage of air into the internal bellows triggers the carriage which holds the paper. The carriage moves from left to right in 6 seconds and then stops. The normal subject will have expired fully within 4 seconds, as will a well-controlled asthmatic, but anyone with a severe degree of obstruction will still be exhaling, with the paper stationary for perhaps 10–15 seconds or until the next breath must be taken. Some machines provide a print-out of the volume measurement, with a correction for ambient temperature, and some have the facility to compare the results with mean predicted levels for a person of that age, height and sex. A normal tracing is shown in Fig. 5.4, *see* page 61; tracings from an asthmatic subject before (i) and after (ii) the inhalation of a beta$_2$-agonist, salbutamol, are shown in Fig. 5.5, *see* page 62.

Many measurements may be taken from a spirometer tracing, but none have greater value than the FEV_1 and the FVC (measured in litres). The FEV_1 and the PEFR usually behave similarly, because both reflect flow in the larger divisions of the pulmonary airways. However, on occasions the observer may be misled by a return to normal of the PEFR after an exacerbation of asthma. The FVC may still be reduced, due to residual obstruction of the smaller calibre bronchioles (which contribute proportionately little to the PEFR result) which leads to peripheral air-trapping and a reduction in the FVC. The low FVC is associated with a raised residual volume (Fig. 5.6, *see* page 64). Thus, the spirometer may contribute useful additional information.

As explained earlier, airflow may be reduced by:

1 events in the bronchus itself, such as bronchoconstriction, mucosal oedema and mucus hypersecretion;
2 pressure on the airways from air trapped in alveoli during forced expiration.

The latter occurs when increasing expiratory pressure cannot expel air at a faster rate and indeed it serves only to compress the bronchi and bronchioles, thereby worsening the situation. On such occasions, more gentle expiration results in a paradoxical improvement in flow rate characteristics (Fig. 5.7). Care needs to be taken on such occasions because this variability might be attributed to the benefits of therapy.

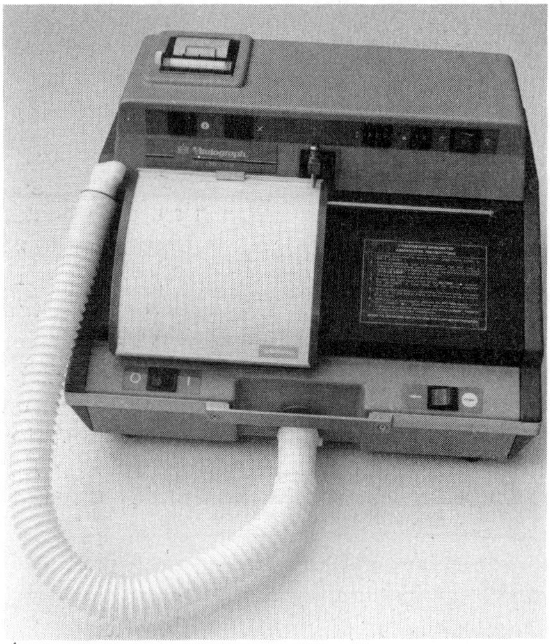

(a) Vitalograph dry bellows spirometer

(b) Vitalograph Compact spirometer with pneumotachograph

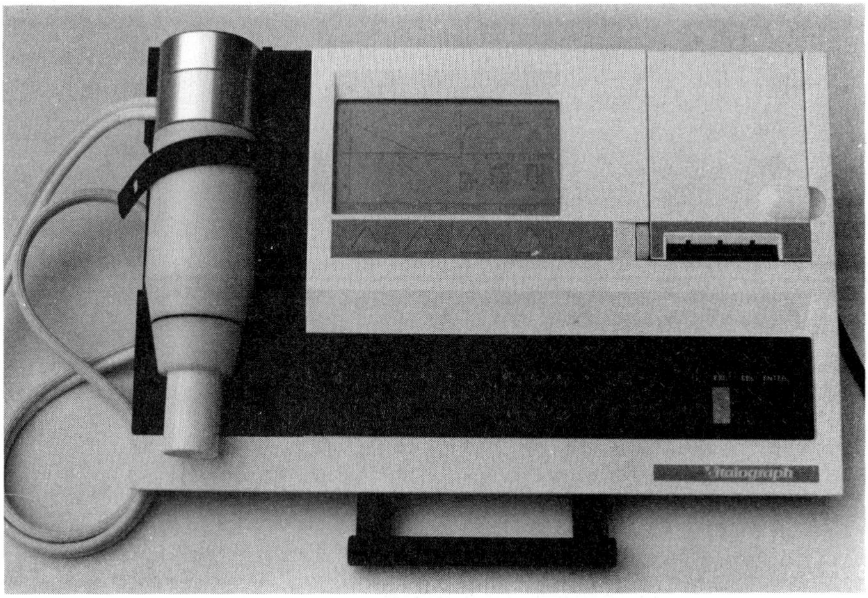

Figure 5.3 Vitalograph devices.

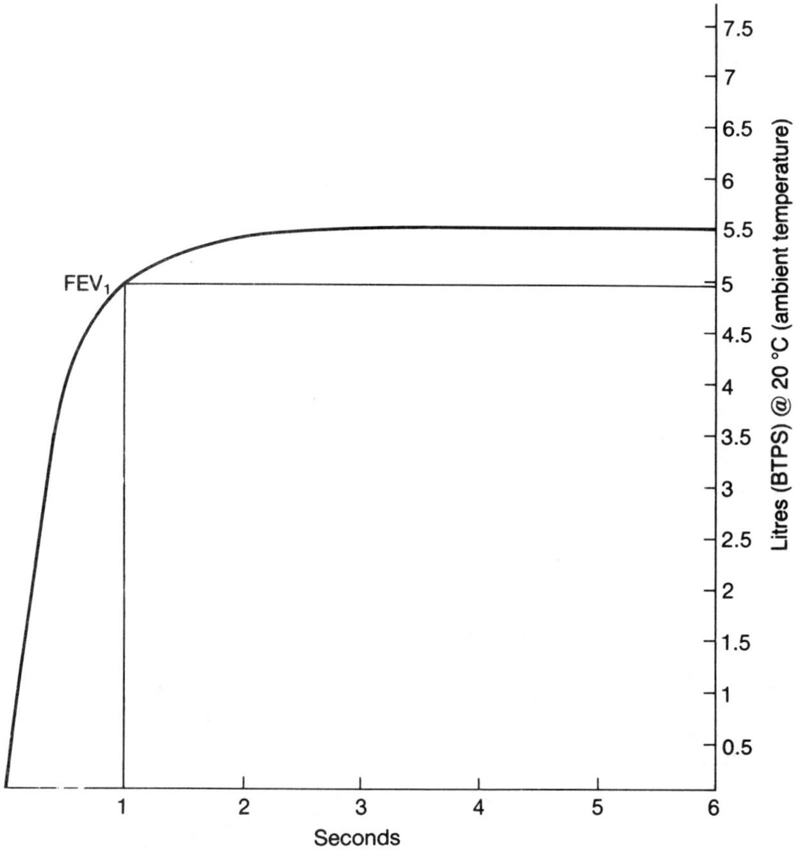

Figure 5.4 Normal spirometry trace (spirogram).

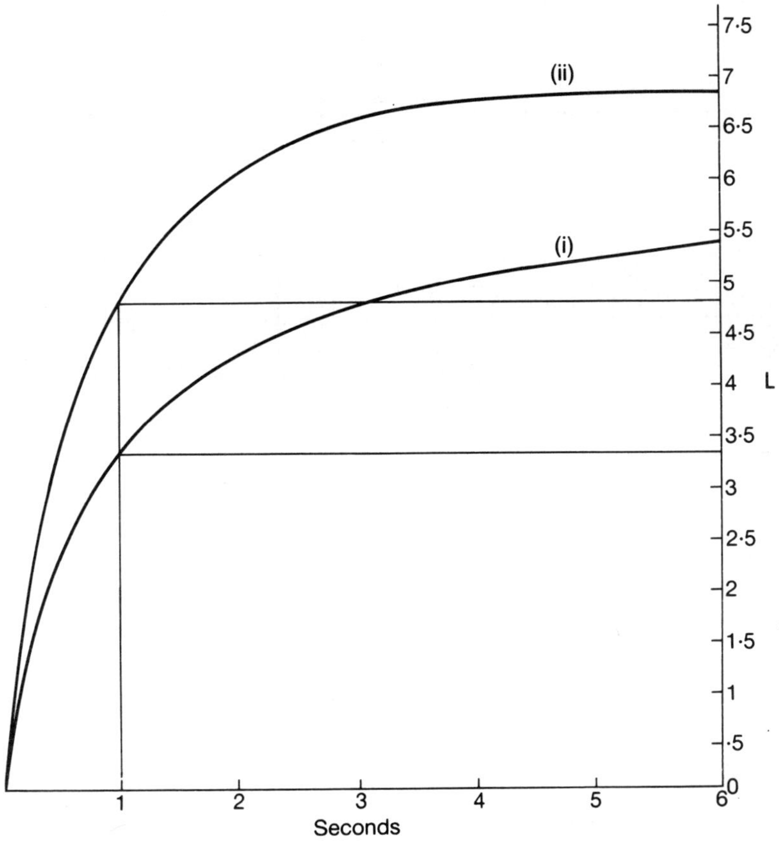

Figure 5.5 Spirometry in 30 year old 6′2″ male asthmatic, (i) before and (ii) after inhalation of 2 puffs of salbutamol inhaler.

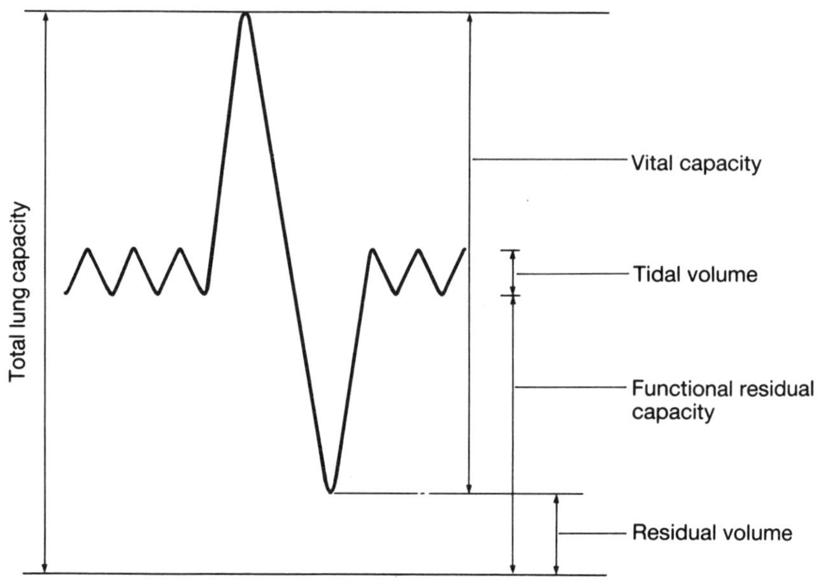

Figure 5.6 Lung volumes.

Method

1. Calibrate the equipment (to room temperature, patient's height, age and sex).
2. Ensure that the paper is correctly positioned and that the pointer is accurately located on the starting point.
3. Instruct the patient to take as deep a breath as is possible.
4. Insert the mouthpiece between the lips and seal them.
5. The patient should breathe out as hard and as completely as possible.
6. The patient should not stop breathing out until the carriage has stopped and the pointer has stopped rising—this is the FVC.

Measurements may be made from the paper or retrieved from the device itself.

Care must be taken with some middle-aged and elderly patients, especially those who have severe degrees of airflow limitation and perhaps some vertebrobasilar insufficiency, because they may suffer sudden, acute syncope or a drop-attack during the course of a prolonged forced expiration. Recovery is rapid, but the effect on the patient is distressing.

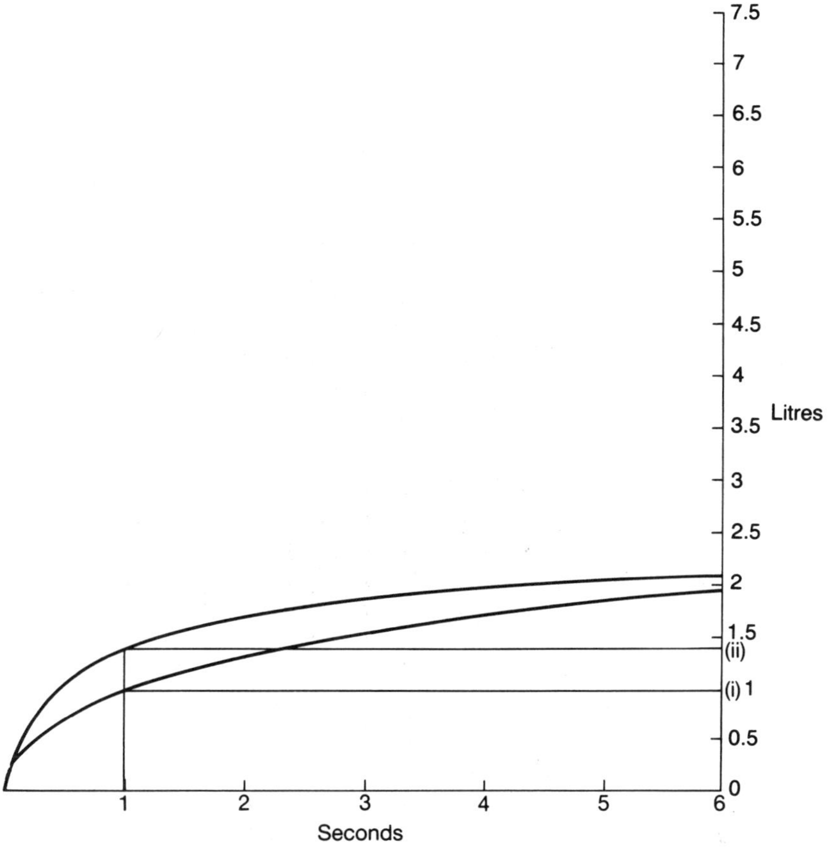

Figure 5.7 Paradoxical rise in FEV_1 (ii) with gentle vs forced (i) expiration (air-trapping and 'floppy' tubes).

Source of error

1 Failure of patient to take an adequate breath.
2 Failure of patient to seal the lips.
3 Problems with the shape of the mouthpiece, false teeth, etc.
4 Escape of air down the patient's nose.
5 Slow start to the expiration, giving a sigmoid curve (Fig. 5.8).
6 Failure of patient to maintain forced expiration, thereby allowing air to leak.
7 Patient breathing in through the nose during the procedure and adding this to the expired total (Fig. 5.9, *see* page 67).

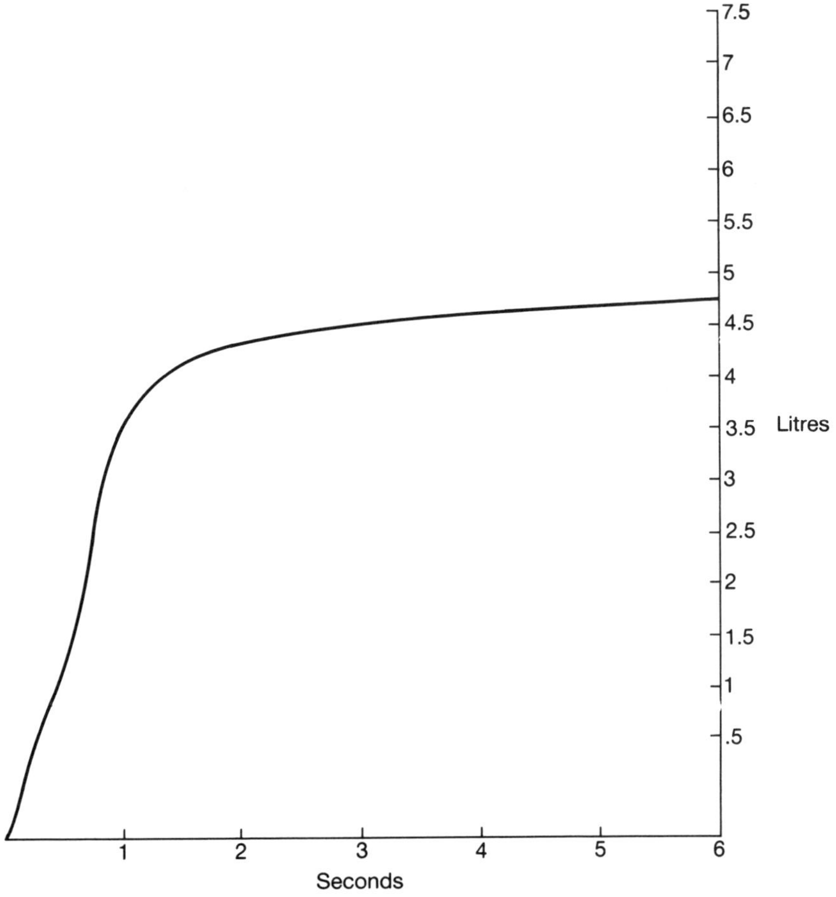

Figure 5.8 Sigmoid curve of slow start to forced expiration

In asthma the FEV_1 is reduced, especially in relation to the FVC, although the latter may also be reduced, as a reflection of increased resistance in the smaller airways. Normally, the FEV_1 represents 75% or more of the FVC, but simple ratios or percentages may be misleading—the ratio may be maintained but both FEV_1 and FVC may be much reduced. Diseases of the lung parenchyma, compared with those of the bronchial tree, result in an overall reduction of volumes.

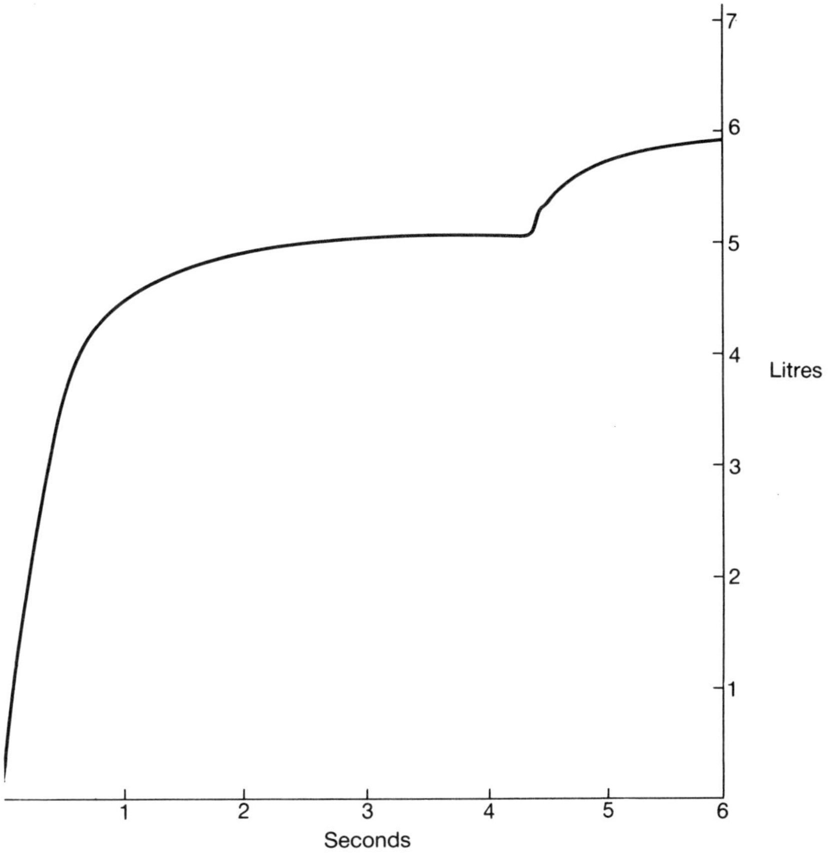

Figure 5.9 Gross example of consequences of taking a nasal breath during FVC procedure thus adding to final volume – only obvious with a visual spirogram.

Flow-volume measurements

Plotting expiratory flow against the volume of air expired produces a flow–volume curve. The normal curve shows a rapid rise in flow rate to the PEFR followed by a slow linear decline to zero at the point at which the FVC has been exhaled and only the residual volume remains.

Narrowing of the airways, due to changes in their walls, results in a lower PEFR and an initially faster drop in flow rate as the lungs empty (Fig. 5.10).

During forced expiration in patients with emphysema, and loss of elasticity of the supporting tissue in the lungs, the bronchi are not supported and they narrow quickly. The initial expiratory flow is rapid but then it falls as pleural and alveolar pressures compress the bronchi, restricting expiratory flow to a very low rate that is almost constant (Fig. 5.11).

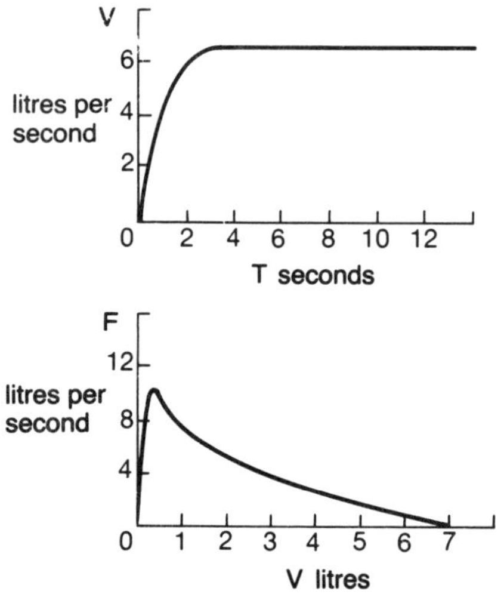

Figure 5.10 Parallel recordings of spirogram and flow-volume curve in asthma.

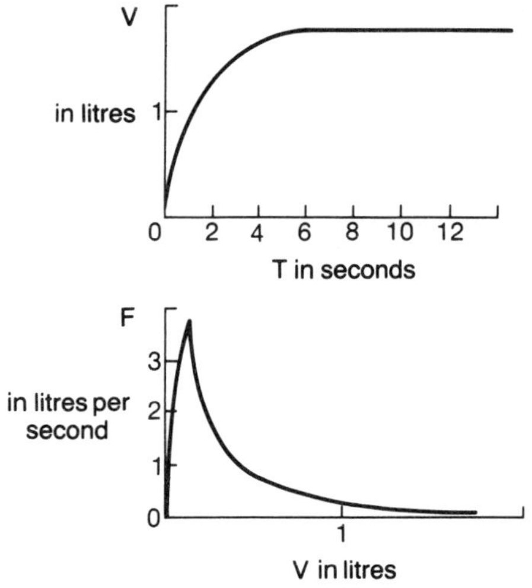

Figure 5.11 Parallel recordings of spirogram and flow-volume curve in emphysema ('floppy tubes').

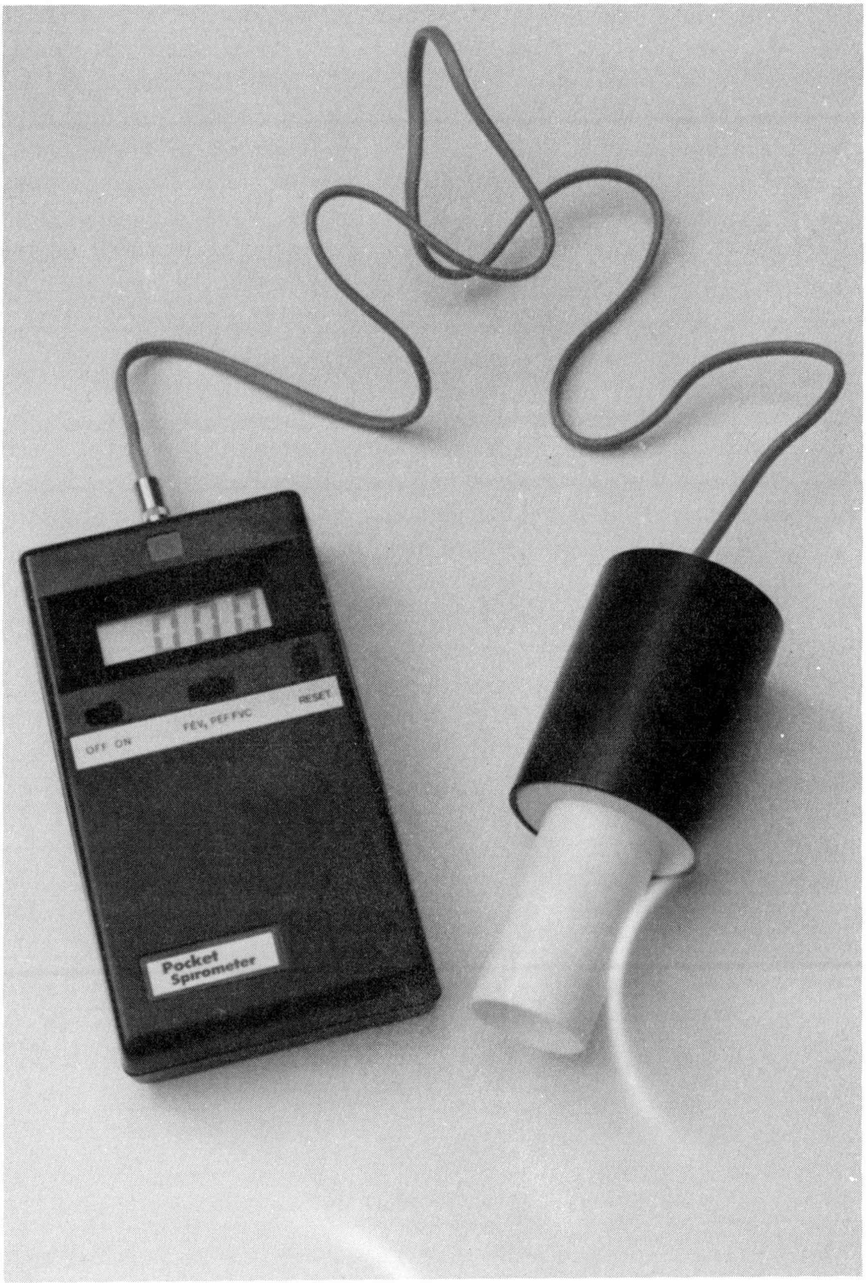

Figure 5.12 Pocket Spirometer.

Dry-bellows devices, such as the Vitalograph, have replaced the wet-spirometer and kymograph for simple spirometry. They are accurate (±2%) but heavy and bulky. More portable devices are now available which work on different principles (Fig. 5.12). For example, the Pocket Spirometer is cheap and measures PEFR, FEV_1 and FVC, although it has no visual image of the spirogram. Forced expiration through the mouthpiece holder unit rotates a very light vane whose movement is measured by an optical system. The flow is then integrated electronically to provide the volume measurements. I find that the shape of the spirogram provides useful information, which can be used partly to check on the consistency of patient effort; a slight drawback is that the vane does not move in very slow airstreams such as those found in a patient with severe obstruction.

The Vitalograph Compact (Fig. 5.3b, *see* page 61), accurate to ±3%, uses a hand-held pneumotachograph. A pneumotachograph measures the pressure-drop across a fine gauge mesh interposed in the air current which is converted into an electrical signal by a transducer. This signal is indicative of 'flow' (Fig. 5.13). The volume figures are obtained by integrating the flow rate. The pneumotachograph of the Compact allows the measurement of inspiratory variables and the construction of a flow–volume loop.

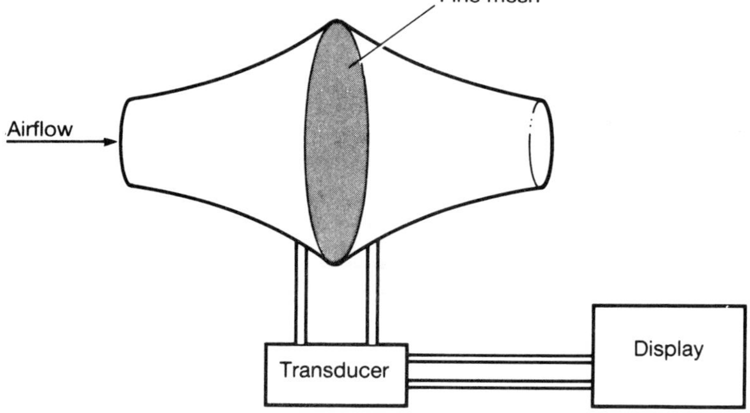

Figure 5.13 Pneumotachograph.

Diagnostic and therapeutic tests

Apart from making solitary PEFR and spirometry readings, all of these pieces of equipment can be used in the following diagnostic and therapeutic tests.

The exercise test

The exercise test is a safe form of provocative manoeuvre, which can be performed with the minimum of equipment. During and after exercise, the non-asthmatic will show little change in airflow characteristics except for a transient bronchodilatation. Most people will probably be 'puffed out', and breathless after vigorous exercise, but they will not experience bronchoconstriction.

In the absence of treatment, most asthmatics show evidence of airflow limitation in response to exercise, with a fall in PEFR or FEV_1, which is maximal at between 3 and 7 minutes after exercise. A fall of 15% is accepted as being diagnostic of exercise-induced asthma. The exercise test can be used diagnostically or to assess the efficacy of therapeutic agents in preventing exercise-induced asthma.

Method

1 Measure resting PEFR or FEV_1.
2 The patient should take 6 minutes' vigorous exercise, e.g. running.
3 Measure PEFR immediately upon completion of exercise.
4 Measure PEFR every 2 minutes up to 10 minutes after the completion of exercise.

When a drop in PEFR has occurred, it can be demonstrably reversed with an inhaled $beta_2$-agonist.

More formal exercise tests are performed in hospital or research establishments. These include heart-rate monitoring and graded levels of exercise on a treadmill. At the other extreme, patients can perform their own exercise tests under everyday conditions if they take a peak-flow meter with them to the sports field, for example. Indeed, this may be the only way to detect exercise-induced asthma when the conditions of exercise are difficult to reproduce artificially.

Reversibility tests

Reversibility tests are designed to detect and measure any improvement in reduced bronchial airflow, in response to anti-asthma therapy. Such tests are not confined to the assessment of the effects of bronchodilators, as is commonly supposed, but they cover the range of inhaled $beta_2$-agonists, anticholinergics and oral corticosteroids. The time course of the test will change with the therapeutic agent used. The tests may be considered to be both diagnostic and trials of therapy. A rise of 15% is significant.

Methods

$Beta_2$-agonists

1 Measure PEFR/spirometry.
2 The patient should be given a $beta_2$-agonist, e.g. salbutamol, to inhale via an aerosol inhaler, dry powder device or nebulizer.
3 Measure PEFR/spirometry after 15 minutes.

Anticholinergics

1 Measure PEFR/spirometry.
2 The patient should be given an anticholinergic, e.g. ipratropium, to inhale via an aerosol or nebulizer.
3 Measure PEFR/spirometry after 30 – 45 minutes.

Steroid trial

When the response to bronchodilator therapy is inadequate with evidence of persistent airflow limitation, a steroid trial should be carried out. Oral prednisolone, in a dosage of 0.6 mg/kg bodyweight/day, is administered as a single daily dose after breakfast, for 2 weeks. A typical dosage is 30 – 40 mg.

Occasionally, the benefits of therapy are too subtle to be demonstrated by relatively simple tests, such as spirometry or PEFR measurement. However, they may be represented by a functional improvement which will be reflected in improved exercise tolerance.

In those patients with severely limited respiratory function tests, which perhaps reflect a marked degree of irreversible obstruction or emphysema, a 12-minute walking test may be appropriate. The distance walked in 12 minutes is measured before and after therapy.

Another difficult situation is assessment of intermittent symptoms in small children, who are too young to carry out simple respiratory function tests. Assessment will depend upon the child's symptoms and physical signs (if present) and the clinical response to treatment, for example, by observation of activities and nocturnal disturbances.

Caution

It is necessary to sound a cautionary note about provocation tests. It may appear to be very attractive to implicate an inhaled allergen by proving its role in provoking clinical asthma. The severity of the response is impossible to predict, but it can result in a marked early asthmatic response, followed by a severe late response. Such tests should be performed only in respiratory units where there are resuscitation facilities immediately to hand. When carried out in the surgery, the early response may take the GP by surprise; the late response may begin after the patient has gone home and it may reach its peak during the night.

6 Anti-asthma Drugs

History – Bronchodilators – $Beta_2$-adrenergic stimulants – Anticholinergics – Theophyllines – Corticosteroids – Sodium cromoglycate – Nedocromil sodium – Ketotifen – Side effects – Monitor growth in children – Beware oral before giving i.v. theophylline – Metabolism of theophylline varies – Trade names

The improvements in the management of asthma since 1970 are largely the result of the introduction of new drugs and the accumulation of experience in how best to use them.

Some drugs have been available for decades but their application has changed as a result of new pharmaceutical technology, concern about safety margins and their displacement by new preparations. Take, for example, the methylxanthines, such as theophylline. Gastrointestinal symptoms, in particular, limited their use when taken orally and they were used predominantly by rectal suppository or intravenous injection. However, new oral slow-release preparations have increased their clinical use so much so that when intravenous administration is required for the treatment of severe asthma there is the risk of overdosage due to the presence of indeterminate amounts of previously ingested oral preparations. An estimation of serum theophylline levels is mandatory before intravenous injection.

Adrenaline and isoprenaline increased in popularity when they became available in metered-dose aerosols. These preparations, with their advantage of rapid onset of action, were sold over the counter without prescription. However, by the mid 1960s, concern was expressed over the rise in asthma deaths, particularly in the young; this rise was paralleled by the increasing sales of over the counter aerosols. These extra deaths probably resulted from a combination of factors.

1 Unlimited, uncontrolled use of powerful pharmacological agents, with inadequate medical guidance and supervision.
2 Failure to receive appropriate additional therapy, such as corticosteroids, as asthmatic symptoms became less responsive to the inhaled bronchodilators.

3 Possible dysrhythmias caused by high levels of adrenaline or isoprenaline in the presence of hypoxaemia.
4 Possible adverse reactions to aerosol propellants.

These problems led to the introduction of more selective beta_2-agonist bronchodilators, which are safer, but these are available only on prescription whereas the entire range of methylxanthines and a selection of mixtures for inhalation, containing combinations of adrenaline, atropine and papaverine, are still available over the counter.

When considering the actions of anti-asthma drugs, it is convenient to divide them into groups as follows.

1 Bronchodilators:
   i beta_2-adrenergic stimulants, e.g. salbutamol;
   ii anticholinergics, e.g. ipratropium;
   iii theophyllines (*see* item 4).
2 Corticosteroids:
   i systemic, e.g. prednisolone;
   ii inhaled, e.g. beclomethasone.
3 Non-steroidal inhaled prophylactics:
   i sodium cromoglycate;
   ii nedocromil sodium.
4 Methylxanthines, e.g. theophylline.
5 Oral prophylactics, e.g. ketotifen.

Bronchodilators

Bronchodilators work by relaxing contracted bronchial smooth muscle.

Beta_2-agonists

Sympathetic receptors have been divided into alpha- and beta-receptors, the beta-receptors being further subdivided into beta_1- and beta_2-receptors according to their site and their specific action (Fig. 6.1). For our purposes we can consider beta_1-receptors as being in the heart and beta_2-receptors in the bronchi, where their stimulation leads to bronchodilatation. Beta_2-stimulants are not absolutely specific to the lungs and they do have a dose-dependent effect on receptors in both the heart and voluntary muscle, leading to tachycardia and tremor.

		Alpha	Beta	
			Beta$_1$ (heart)	Beta$_2$ (bronchi)
Naturally occurring	Noradrenaline	✓		
	Adrenaline	✓	✓	✓
Synthetic	Isoprenaline		✓	✓
	Orciprenaline		△	✓
	Salbutamol			✓

Key
✓ Yes
△ Partial response

Figure 6.1 Sympathetic receptors and their responses.

Beta$_2$-agonists (such as salbutamol, terbutaline, fenoterol and reproterol) are the most commonly prescribed anti-asthma drugs in clinical use in the United Kingdom. All beta$_2$-agonists are similar in their therapeutic effects, with a rapid onset of action reaching its maximum in 5 – 15 minutes. There are small differences in their duration of action, their half-lives after inhalation varying between 3 and 8 hours. It is essential for the GP to be familiar with one or two of these agents which, through a variety of modes of delivery, will cover most situations.

Beta$_2$-agonists have displaced adrenaline and isoprenaline as therapeutic agents for reasons of safety. Their advantages lie in their rapid onset of action and in their well-proven margin of safety. However, this rapid response, which can be experienced by the patient and measured objectively, has often meant that patients and doctors have tended to tackle poor control simply by switching from one beta$_2$-stimulant to another. Unfortunately, some patients who feel better let their prophylactic therapy lapse, only to substitute it with the ever-increasing administration of inhaled bronchodilators.

What is the role of the beta$_2$-stimulant?

1 To reverse increased airways resistance due to bronchoconstriction triggered by exercise or allergic insult.
2 As a prophylactic to prevent exercise-induced asthma, partly through its mast cell stabilizing properties.
3 To enhance mucociliary clearance which may be useful in both asthma and bronchiectasis.

They have no effect on the inflammatory processes which lead to bronchial hyperreactivity and mucosal oedema. The introduction of nebulizers has led patients and doctors to believe that if a modest dose is ineffective then it should be increased. This is not the case. The only means of reversing a significant degree of mucosal oedema and mucus production is by administering systemic corticosteroids. Rising dosage requirements should be seen as an indication that additional therapy is required, not more of the same.

Dosage and means of administration

The dosage and the dose interval depend on the individual, the clinical circumstances and the route of administration. As larger doses are used, especially with oral or nebulizer administration, so side effects are more common (Fig. 6.2), although some tolerance does develop.

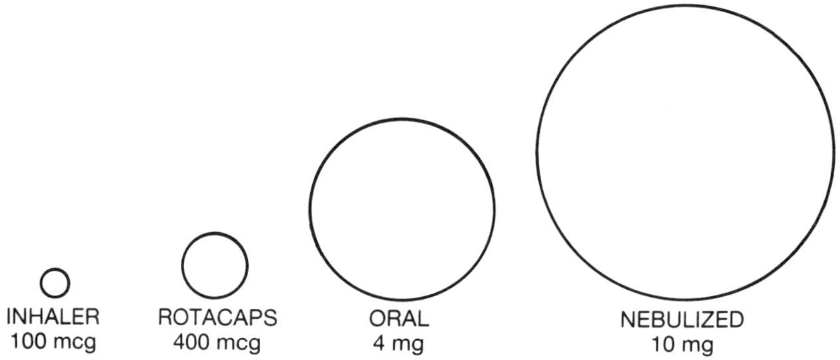

Figure 6.2 Relative doses of beta$_2$-agonists depending on means of administration.

Using salbutamol as an example, typical doses are as follows.

Aerosol inhaler:

100 μg/puff, 1 or 2 puffs every 4–6 hours.

Dry powder device:

400 (or 200) μg one or more doses every 4–6 hours.

Respirator solution (nebulizer):

(a) 5 mg/ml in 20 ml bottles—up to 10 mg diluted to 2–4 ml with sterile physiological saline, every 4 hours or as required;
(b) 2.5 or 5 mg in 2.5 ml Nebules every 4 hours or depending on need (preservative-free).

Oral route:

syrup 2 mg/5 ml or tablets 2 mg, 4 mg every 6 hours; sustained-release tablets, 4 mg or 8 mg every 12 hours.

Subcutaneous/intramuscular injection:

500 μg/1 ml, 8 μg/kg every 4 hours.

Slow intravenous injection:

250 μg/5 ml (4 μg/kg) as required.

Side effects

The type and severity of side effects vary with dosage and from patient to patient. Tremor, muscle cramps, tachycardia and nervousness can all occur. High doses may precipitate angina pectoris and dysrhythmias, especially in elderly patients who have ischaemic heart disease.

The use of nebulized $beta_2$-stimulants in infants may lead to clinical deterioration. Even if the solution is initially isotonic, it will tend to become hypertonic during nebulization, due to water evaporation from the tiny droplets. Hypertonic and hypotonic solutions may precipitate bronchial smooth muscle contraction and, in infants under 15 months, there is no consistent response to $beta_2$-stimulants.

Rimiterol (Pulmadil, not to be confused with Pulmicort) has a very short duration of action which makes it unsuitable as a clinical therapeutic agent. However, it is useful for reversibility testing.

Anticholinergics

Anticholinergics block the vagal cholinergic receptors in the bronchial wall, leading to bronchodilatation if there is vagally induced bronchoconstriction. The only drug from this group that is in regular use in the United Kingdom is ipratropium bromide, which has a latent period of 30 – 45 minutes. It is thought to have little adverse effect on ciliary activity or in altering bronchial mucus, although it does occasionally appear to contribute to thickening of the mucus.

Ipratropium tends to be used in older patients (particularly those with 'chronic bronchitis'), perhaps because of greater reactivity of the cholinergic over the adrenergic receptors in middle aged and older patients. Certainly, some patients do exhibit a greater response to a combination of anti-cholinergic and $beta_2$-stimulants than to either agent taken alone. However, it has been found that 40% of infantile asthmatics will respond to ipratropium at a stage when they show no response to $beta_2$-agonists; it is not possible to predict which infants will respond in this way.

Before regular use of anticholinergics, it is worth performing a specific reversibility test; after inhalation an interval of 30 – 45 minutes should be left before measuring the patient's response.

Dosage and means of administration

Aerosol inhaler:

18 μg/puff, 1 – 2 puffs 4 times daily.

Forte aerosol inhaler:

36 μg/puff, 1 – 2 puffs 4 times daily.

Nebulizer solution:

250 μg/ml in 2 ml unit dose vials, dose 100 – 500 μg, diluted to 3 ml with sterile physiological saline.

Side effects

The side effects of anticholinergics are dosage-dependent and therefore they are more common after nebulizer therapy. Dry mouth, blurred vision, urinary retention and constipation may occur, and care must be taken when using nebulized ipratropium via a mask in patients with glaucoma. Clinical deterioration after using nebulized ipratroprium was recognized quite early, presumably because of the longer latent period before its therapeutic effect became apparent. The reaction was related to:

1 hypotonic solution;
2 specific sensitivity to the bromide moiety;
3 reaction to the preservatives in the preparation.

However, the solution is now isotonic, with instructions to dilute with physiological saline, and current preparations are preservative-free.

Corticosteroids

The mechanism of action of corticosteroids in asthma is not clearly understood. Corticosteroids appear to enhance the sensitivity and to maintain the number of beta$_2$-adrenergic receptors on bronchial smooth muscle cells. More importantly, they exert a powerful anti-inflammatory effect, with a consequent reduction in mucosal oedema, mucus hypersecretion and bronchial hyperreactivity. The observation that corticosteroids disperse congregated eosinophils is related to this action.

The ability of corticosteroids to direct cells to produce macrocortin (lipomodulin) might be central to their mechanism of action. Macrocortin inhibits phospholipase A_2, the effects of which will be far-reaching because the production of leukotrienes, prostaglandins and chemotactic factors will be inhibited and the degranulation of the mast cells will be limited.

Short term (hours) pre-treatment with corticosteroids blocks only the late asthmatic response; treatment for longer periods (weeks) will reduce the early response, although it will not *block* the early response in the same way that sodium cromoglycate and nedocromil sodium block it.

Systemic corticosteroids

Corticosteroids have been used in the treatment of asthma since 1950. Despite the initial euphoria surrounding their use, extreme caution is now exercised in the prescription of these drugs following their association with serious side effects if used for a prolonged period in moderate dosage. Even today, with other anti-asthma agents now available, it may be difficult to balance the benefits of long term corticosteroid therapy against the side effects for a severe asthmatic and the compromise is often unsatisfactory.

However, when used judiciously, the effects of corticosteroids are often dramatic and almost always beneficial. The most commonly prescribed oral steroid in the United Kingdom is prednisolone, because it has a better activity/side effect profile than other corticosteroids. Prednisone is less often prescribed, mainly because it has to be converted to prednisolone in the liver before it becomes active. ACTH is less satisfactory as it depends upon the patient's adrenal cortex for its effect and also because there is a parallel mineralocorticoid effect which causes greater salt and water retention. It is important to use an adequate dosage of systemic corticosteroids for a sufficient length of time to achieve the desired effect. When the patient's condition has stabilized, it is possible to decide whether to stop the corticosteroids abruptly, tail them off gradually or to replace them with an inhaled prophylactic agent. The inflammatory process must be totally suppressed before withdrawal or transfer to an inhaled prophylactic, otherwise inflammation will slowly recur and perhaps lead to the prescription of repeated inadequate short courses of systemic steroids, which is not uncommon.

Dosage and preparations

An effective dose in an adult will be between 30 and 60 mg of prednisolone—0.6 mg/kg body weight offers the best compromise between the greatest efficacy and least side effects. In children, the dosage is set, arbitrarily, at 1 – 2 mg/kg/day. The plasma half-life of prednisolone is 2 – 3 hours and its biological half-life is 24 – 36 hours, which make it suitable for administration once daily, after breakfast. A single dose not only has a greater pharmacological effect but is also more 'physiological' in that it is superimposed upon the body's normal adrenocortical surge in the morning, making it less likely to upset the body's diurnal rhythm. For a small number of patients a split dose administered twice daily is preferred.

The administration of corticosteroids is attended by a latent period before any therapeutic effects are apparent; a maximum effect is observed at 9 – 10 hours with oral prednisolone and at 7 – 8 hours with intravenous hydrocortisone. Only in the most severe cases of acute asthma is the intravenous route indicated, unless the patient is vomiting. When hydrocortisone is used, it should be reconstituted by dissolving hydrocortisone sodium succinate powder in sterile water for injection. The sodium phosphate preparation may appear to be more convenient because it is already dissolved, but its intravenous injection can cause very distressing intense perineal pruritus, which is not conducive to hastening a patient's recovery.

Prednisolone

Tablets:

1 mg and 5 mg; soluble form Prednesol 5 mg for children and those who find difficulty in swallowing tablets.

Enteric-coated tablets:

2.5 mg and 5 mg; to minimize the risk of indigestion and peptic ulceration.

Side effects

Side effects depend upon dosage, duration of therapy, individual susceptibility, age and body mass. Mental changes, from euphoria to depression, may occur quite quickly, but other side effects become more marked with time: iatrogenic Cushing's disease, osteoporosis, hypertension, hyperglycaemia, peptic ulceration, salt and water retention, cataracts, purpura, acne, hypokalaemia, muscle weakness and wasting, thinning of the skin and adrenal suppression.

The prolonged use of systemic corticosteroids may suppress growth in children; growth suppression is less common if an alternate day regimen is adopted. ACTH may work by stimulating the body's own adrenal glands but an effective dosage will not be without side effects.

Inhaled corticosteroids

The advent of inhaled corticosteroids, which work by virtue of their high surface activity, has extended the valuable contribution and benefits of corticosteroid therapy to many more asthma sufferers. Their mode of action is the same as that for systemic corticosteroids, but there is a period of

3 – 7 days before they are fully effective depending upon the level of bronchial inflammatory activity at the time of their introduction.

As doses administered are very small, inhaled steroids should not be used to treat severe exacerbations of asthma. It is not unknown for a patient whose asthma was previously well controlled on a typical dosage to suffer a breakthrough of symptoms and to have the dosage of inhaled steroid increased to high but ineffective levels; in such a case, the immediate introduction of oral prednisolone would have resolved the problem quickly.

Owing to the surface activity of these drugs (such as beclomethasone), there is little risk of systemic side effects from gastrointestinal absorption. Inactivation is rapid on first pass through the liver, unless the dosage exceeds the threshold. Despite this, a higher proportion of beclomethasone in the blood will have been absorbed from the bronchial tree.

The dosage of inhaled steroid necessary to bring about either demonstrable suppression of the pituitary – adrenal axis or evidence of systemic side effects will depend upon the age, sex and size of the patient and upon individual sensitivity. The inhalation of 1000 – 1600 μg of beclomethasone dipropionate has biochemically detectable effects in an adult but these and lower doses may be associated with purpura in some patients. Although doses of up to 600 μg of beclomethasone dipropionate have been shown to have no adverse effect on children's growth, the prescriber must be vigilant and monitor every child's growth during the course of their asthma treatment. Dry powder preparations of beclomethasone diproprionate will commonly use 800 μg daily and this would appear to be safe.

In the event of serious, intercurrent illness, undergoing surgical procedures or suffering an accident, patients who are taking 1500 μg or more of beclomethasone dipropionate should be treated as if they were on systemic corticosteroids and it might be wise for them to carry a steroid card. High-dose preparations, such as Becloforte, should be reserved for cases of severe asthma and not to compensate for undertreatment resulting from the use of conventional dosages administered with poorly-taught inhaler techniques. It is essential to gain the maximum effect from the minimum dosage.

Beclomethasone dipropionate for use in a nebulizer is produced as an aqueous suspension. Although useful in infants and small children, it is not often used in adults due to the large volumes required. A solution of budesonide, not yet available for prescription, is said to be more active than the aqueous suspension of beclomethasone dipropionate.

Dosage and means of administration

The three inhaled corticosteroids available in the United Kingdom are beclomethasone dipropionate, betamethasone and budesonide. When first introduced, the inhaled steroids were administered on a 4 times a day regimen, but this has subsequently been shown to be unnecessary. Twice daily administration is adequate and convenient and meets with far greater compliance from the patient who has fewer instructions to remember. Some patients on higher dosages may report greater benefit when the dosage is divided into 3 or 4 doses. Typical dosages for inhaled corticosteroids using beclomethasone as an example.

Aerosol inhaler:

50, 100, 250 μg/puff; typical adult dose 200 μg twice daily.

Dry powder:

100, 200, 400 μg; typical adult dose 400 μg twice daily.

Suspension:

50 μg/ml; perhaps 100 μg (2 ml), 2 – 4 times daily; 10 ml bottle.

Side effects

The only common side effects of inhaled corticosteroids are oropharyngeal thrush and hoarseness of the voice. Thrush is characteristic, with reddening of the mucosa, overlain with adherent white plaques. It tends to recur in the same patients, despite general precautions, such as taking a drink after inhalation to wash out the mouth and the throat, but it does respond to treatment with topical antifungal agents, such as nystatin or amphotericin given as lozenges or oral suspension. Hoarseness or dysphonia may be caused by reversible laryngeal muscle atrophy related to steroid inhalation. Systemic side effects are dosage-dependent; purpura and osteoporosis should be considered in menopausal patients and a possible increase in cataracts in others.

Non-steroidal inhaled prophylactic agents

Sodium cromoglycate

Sodium cromoglycate was introduced in 1968. Its development was a departure from the established therapeutic agents for asthma, such as the bronchodilators and systemic corticosteroids, in that it worked purely as a prophylactic agent. This approach allowed a reduction in dosages of inhaled bronchodilators and systemic corticosteroids. Sodium cromoglycate's novel mode of action, in stabilizing mast cell membranes, thereby preventing degranulation and the release of pre-formed mediators, added great impetus to the investigation of the underlying mechanisms of asthma. However, its mode of action is far more complex than was at first thought; it is now known that it blocks both the early and late asthmatic responses and prevents exercise-induced asthma if taken in advance. Typically, sodium cromoglycate is taken 4 times a day as a preventive, but it may be necessary to increase the frequency if the challenge is great.

It is important to distinguish between the time taken to suppress the inflammatory reaction that leads to bronchial hyperreactivity, which may be up to 6 weeks, and the immediate blockade of exercise-induced asthma, when sodium cromoglycate is inhaled a few minutes before exercise is taken.

Dosage and means of administration

The initial preparation was a dry powder Spincap, which had the immediate advantage of requiring no co-ordination, simply inspiratory effort. Now for added convenience and for those who have good hand–breath co-ordination, a metered-dose aerosol inhaler is available. For the very young, a nebulizer solution is produced.

Aerosol inhaler:

5 mg/puff, 1 – 2 puffs, 4 times daily.

Dry-powder:

20 mg Spincap, 4 times daily.

Nebulizer solution:

10 mg/ml as 2 ml ampoules; 2 ml 4 times daily.

Side effects

No serious side effects of sodium cromoglycate are known. The only troublesome problem which some patients have found with the dry powder preparation is that it might induce coughing which in turn might lead to wheezing. To obviate this problem, the initial preparation contained isoprenaline 0.1 mg (Intal Compound). Unfortunately, patients often forget the rationale of their therapy, especially when a 'preventive' also appears to relieve bronchoconstriction so effectively, and this has led to many patients who take Intal Compound using it inappropriately. The vast majority of Intal users take it 'plain' without problems.

Nedocromil sodium

Nedocromil sodium is the most recent addition to the therapeutic armamentarium. It inhibits exercise-induced asthma and both the early and late asthmatic responses to an allergic challenge by inhibiting mediator release from cells in the bronchial mucosa. This includes preformed and membrane-derived mediators, as well as chemotactic factors, thereby reducing the cellular infiltrate. It appears to be more effective than sodium cromoglycate in these respects but it will have to compete with inhaled corticosteroids in the treatment of adult asthma.

As the mechanism of action of nedocromil sodium differs from the mechanism of action of both sodium cromoglycate and inhaled steroids, it is likely that its use and consequent effects will define its particular role in the therapy of asthmatics, bearing in mind that it has taken almost 20 years to evolve our current application of the drugs available hitherto. Nedocromil sodium may be an alternative to low-dose steroids up to 400 μg of beclomethasone dipropionate. Asthma is not an homogeneous clinical entity and I feel that nedocromil sodium will also fulfil a supplementary role in some patients whose asthma is inadequately controlled on higher dosage inhaled steroids. An additional role could be in those asthmatics who suffer from oropharyngeal thrush when given inhaled steroids.

Dosage and means of administration

Nedocromil sodium is available as a metered-dose aerosol inhaler delivering 2 mg per puff. It is recommended that dosage starts at 2 puffs twice daily, but this may be increased to 4 times daily. An effect should be apparent within one week.

Side effects

No important side effects of nedocromil sodium have been reported, but some patients have complained of headaches and others of a bitter taste in the mouth.

Methylxanthines

Theophylline is a dimethylxanthine related to caffeine. It acts primarily as a bronchodilator but in a way that is distinct from the action of beta$_2$-agonists. Its precise mode of action is not understood but it also has stimulatory effects upon the heart and causes diuresis.

Until the development of long-acting slow-release preparations, the role of theophylline was restricted by its significant, subjective side effects. Although absorption is usually good, distribution and particularly elimination are susceptible to change, making it difficult to extrapolate dosages from one patient to another. The metabolism of theophylline is dependent upon a patient's age, diet and smoking habits and is affected by various drugs. It is important to note that the elimination mechanism in the liver is easily saturated and small adjustments may suddenly cause unacceptable toxic side effects.

The clinical use of theophyllines in the United Kingdom is in the treatment of those asthmatics who are taking maximal doses of inhaled beta$_2$-agonists, corticosteroids and, when appropriate, anticholinergics but whose asthma is still not adequately controlled. This applies especially to those patients with nocturnal and morning symptoms in whom theophylline can be a very useful supplementary drug.

Table 6.1

Theophylline clearance reduced by:	Theophylline clearance increased by:
Hepatic disorders	Smoking
Cardiac failure	Alcohol
Erythromycin	Phenytoin
Cimetidine	Phenobarbitone
Allopurinol	Rifampicin
Propranolol	High protein, low carbohydrate diet
Ciprofloxacin	
Oestrogens	
Febrile (viral) illnesses	
Low protein, high carbohydrate diet	
i.e. raised serum concentration	i.e. lower serum concentration

(Theophylline can lower the blood level of lithium in those patients previously stabilized on lithium preparations)

Dosage and means of administration

There is a relation between the serum level of theophylline and its effects, but for safety reasons the best compromise is at serum levels between 10 and 20 μg/ml. It is important to start with modest doses to allow the body to adjust, before increasing the dose to an effective level.

No two theophylline preparations will have the same effect on a patient because each of them possesses different release and absorption characteristics. Irrespective of the differences between individual patients, dosage requirements may vary by up to 5 times to achieve the same blood levels in different patients. It is essential that the prescriber is familiar with the particular preparation being prescribed. If there is any doubt, they should refer to the product data sheet or seek further advice. If a measurement of serum theophylline is made to aid dosage adjustment, it should be taken about 3 – 8 hours after ingestion, depending on the release characteristics of the preparation concerned, and the patient should have been taking a stable dosage for at least 48 hours.

For example, the manufacturer's recommended dosage for Uniphyllin Continus (400 mg—scored tablet) is to take the tablet once daily, starting at 400 mg/day for 1 week, thereafter for those with a body weight of >70 kg to take 800 mg, below 70 kg, 600 mg. It is customary to titrate efficacy against dosage, in the absence of side effects; if benefit is not obtained, the serum theophylline level could be checked. For children, the manufacturer's recommended dose is 9 mg/kg body weight/day, which should be doubled to the nearest 100 mg after 1 week (Uniphyllin paediatric Continus—200 mg, scored tablet). It is important for the prescriber to refer to the product data sheet if he or she is unfamiliar with the preparation.

Side effects

Side effects of theophylline may include restlessness, headache, giddiness, polyuria (enuresis in some children), upper gastrointestinal tract symptoms and diarrhoea. Some children may experience educational problems. High blood levels may be associated with cardiac dysrhythmias, fits and death. This is most likely to occur when:

1 a patient takes tablets inappropriately and at an incorrect dosage;
2 a patient with severe asthma who has already taken a long-acting theophylline then receives an injection of intravenous aminophylline which causes toxic levels that can lead to sudden death.

A strange paradox is that it is possible to purchase theophylline preparations over the counter at a chemist's shop, but not the much safer beta$_2$-agonists. (The author is not advocating the over the counter sale of beta$_2$-agonists but rather the control of theophylline sales.)

Ketotifen

Ketotifen was introduced as an orally active, cromoglycate-like agent. However, it has not been widely adopted in the United Kingdom because it can cause intense drowsiness which may be related to its antihistaminic action.

Dosage and means of administration

Capsules and tablets:

1 mg; 1 or 2, twice daily, starting cautiously to minimize drowsiness.

Elixir:

1 mg/5 ml; 5 ml twice daily.

Side effects

Drowsiness is the most troublesome side effect of ketotifen and may lead to the withdrawal of therapy in individual patients.

Drug combinations

Until recently drug combinations containing ephedrine, theophylline and barbiturates were available; the barbiturate has now been removed. It was present to counteract the restlessness and excitability caused by the ephedrine, which has been largely superseded by more effective drugs.

There are some modern inhaled combinations but, although they may be efficacious in some situations, their use often leads to misinterpretation of their rationale and this should be considered carefully before they are prescribed.

Intal Compound as the dry powder of sodium cromoglycate can provoke coughing and wheezing so isoprenaline was added to the first Spincaps to overcome this problem. Unfortunately, some patients use Intal Compound on demand, rather than prophylactically.

Ventide was introduced as a combination of typical doses of salbutamol and beclomethasone (beta$_2$-agonist and inhaled corticosteroid). This may be convenient if patients do not need extra salbutamol but to have an additional salbutamol inhaler nullifies or negates the concept of the combination inhaler. Encouraging the use of the combination inhaler before exercise or as required both contradicts the rational explanations given to patients and may lead to use on demand.

Duovent is a combination of fenoterol and ipratropium (a beta$_2$-agonist and an anticholinergic) which might be helpful in some patients who need both, but again it lacks the flexibility of being able to vary each of the drug doses individually.

Table 6.2 Trade names of common anti-asthma agents.

Generic name	Proprietary name
	(Not all proprietary ranges are comparable)
Selective beta$_2$-agonists	
Salbutamol	Ventolin, Salbulin, Asmaven, Aerolin Autohaler, Salbuvent, Cobutolin Volmax
Fenoterol	Berotec
Terbutaline	Bricanyl, Monovent
Pirbuterol	Exirel
Reproterol	Bronchodil
Inhaled corticosteroids	
Beclomethasone	Becotide 50, Becotide 100, Becloforte
Betamethasone	Bextasol
Budesonide	Pulmicort, Pulmicort LS
Non-steroidal prophylactic agents	
Sodium cromoglycate	Intal
Nedocromil sodium	Tilade
Ketotifen	Zaditen
Methylxanthines	
Theophylline	*Syrup/liquid:* Biophylline, Nuelin *Tablets*: Nuelin *Sustained-release tablets*: Lasma, Nuelin-SA, Pro-Vent, Sabidal SR, Slo-phyllin, Theo-dur, Theograd, Uniphyllin Continus
Choline theophylline	*Syrup:* Choledyl *Tablet:* Choledyl
Aminophylline	*Tablet:* Phyllocontin Continus-Forte and Paediatric, Pecram *Suppositories:* little used

7 Delivery Systems

Inhaled route preferred – Multiplicity of devices – Match device to patient – 30 per cent cannot use metered dose aerosol inhaler – Compatibility of inhalers with expansion devices – Dry powder devices – Nebulizers – Injections

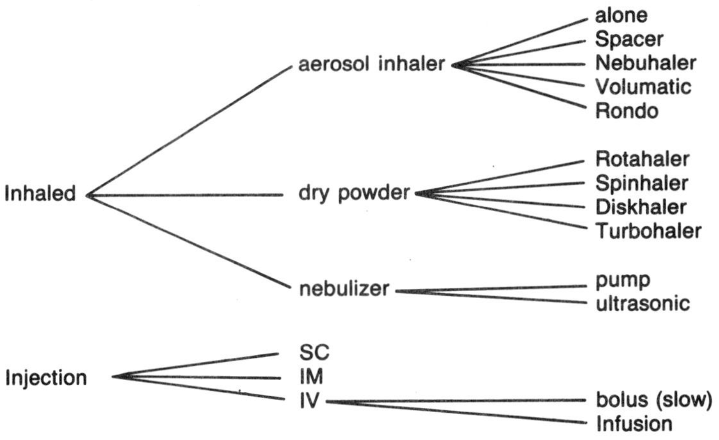

Figure 7.1 Delivery systems.

Oral preparations

IT may appear that the simplest route of administration is by mouth. This may be true in cases in which a genuine systemic approach is necessary, such as with corticosteroids or theophylline. However, the disadvantage of this route of administration is that higher body levels of the drug are required than with direct presentation of the drug to the lungs. As the drug is absorbed from the gut, it enters the hepatic portal system and passes through the liver before reaching the lungs, thus early (first pass) metabolism of the drug takes place. Higher blood and tissue concentrations give rise to a higher incidence of side effects when compared with the same therapeutic effect obtained by inhaled therapy, e.g. $beta_2$-agonists and corticosteroids.

Occasionally oral therapy is the only acceptable route either because of patient preference or a patient's inability to use any inhaling devices except a nebulizer, which may not be appropriate.

Most beta$_2$-stimulants are available as syrups, which are usually sugar-free. Absorption from syrups should be comparable between different preparations but dilution of the basic syrup may upset stability and shorten shelf-life.

Tablet preparations, standard and long-acting or, sustained-release capsules containing multiple pellets, offer considerable scope for altering absorption patterns of drugs. Theophylline preparations are available in a number of tablets and capsules, the effects of which last anything from 6 to 24 hours with considerable variability between patients. Similarly, there are salbutamol preparations designed to last from 6 to 12 hours. Duration of action is not the sole criterion; a consistent, sustained blood level is more important.

Inhaled preparations

Inhalation has become the preferred route of administration for anti-asthma therapy. By this route, provided the drug is in a form that can reach the smallest airways, very small doses of active drugs can be presented to the desired site of action. Even when used properly, any inhalation system allows only 10 – 20% of the available dose to reach the bronchi and bronchioles. However, dosages are calculated so that this is adequate. Inhalation minimizes the risk of systemic side effects and means that drugs are either metabolized locally or absorbed into the bloodstream to be metabolized, usually in the liver. As first pass metabolism by the liver is avoided, the drug's onset of action is considerably faster.

Hand-operated inhalation devices, especially aerosol inhalers, are still looked upon with a mixture of suspicion and fear by some patients and GPs. These images are hard to erase, most notably for GPs because of a possible association with the increase in asthma deaths in the 1960s and for patients because of the notion of being dependent upon the inhaler, relating to the picture of asthma sufferers taking repeated puffs from an inhaler often ineffectively, perhaps because they did not have a demonstration of correct technique. In addition, the original catecholamine inhalers had a short duration of action and so, in the face of unchecked bronchial hyper-reactivity the airways resistance would again rise, necessitating further treatment.

The modern means of inhalation (Fig. 7.2) are shown on the next page.

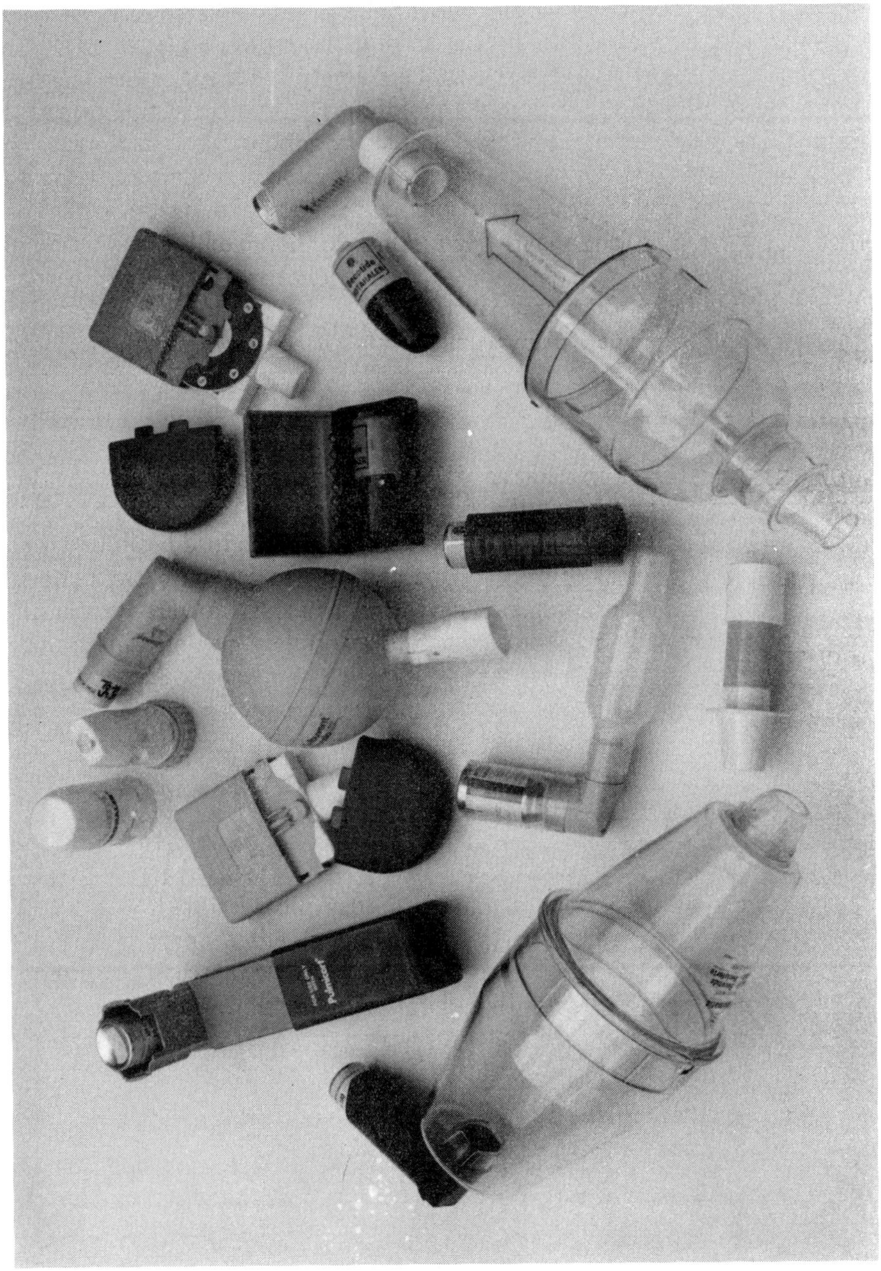

Figure 7.2 A selection of inhaler devices.

Aerosol

The metered-dose aerosol inhaler provides a convenient, very low dosage form of therapy. For example, one 4 mg tablet of salbutamol contains 40 times more of the drug than does one puff of the aerosol inhaler. Metered-dose inhalers are available which contain beta$_2$-agonists, anticholinergics, corticosteroids, sodium cromoglycate or nedocromil sodium. The drug is suspended in a chlorofluorocarbon propellant and the device needs to be gently shaken to suspend the drug evenly before inhalation. A metering valve governs the amount of drug that is released with each discharge.

To use a metered-dose inhaler, it is necessary for the patient to have good hand–breath co-ordination. The first step is to shake the device gently, then, with the mouthpiece between the lips, to trigger the aerosol immediately after the start of inspiration, breathing in smoothly and steadily through the device. The breath is held for 10 seconds before exhaling. The patient should wait for 30 seconds between puffs, to allow the metering valve to re-warm in order to provide consistent dosage.

A recent innovation is the latest version of the Aerolin Autohaler, a metered-dose inhaler containing salbutamol which is breath-activated and easy to set; previous devices were not as easy to use. For some patients however, the force of the aerosol jet against the back of the throat will still inhibit inspiration.

Unfortunately, about 25 – 30% of patients are unable to use a metered-dose inhaler to full effect. Most children below the age of 8 years do not possess the necessary co-ordination. One disadvantage of this form of administration is that the velocity of the aerosol jet can cause excessive deposition of the drug on the back of the mouth and oropharynx. Apart from reducing the amount of drug available for distribution within the lungs, this causes particular problems when corticosteroids are inhaled as their deposition can encourage oral candidiasis (thrush). This side effect occurs in approximately 5% of subjects using inhaled corticosteroids.

Spacer devices and expansion chambers

The Spacer device (Astra) was an early attempt to:

1 reduce the jet effect; and
2 circumvent the problems resulting from poor co-ordination.

This extending box over the mouthpiece of the metered-dose inhaler was clumsy to use, but was compact and helped to a degree. Investigations of inhaled drug distribution in the lungs showed that it tended to be patchy, but if the aerosol discharge could be dispersed in an expansion chamber first, distribution was more even, and also more of the drug entered the lungs.

Thus, the Nebuhaler (Astra) was developed—a 750 ml plastic expansion chamber which housed the metered-dose inhaler at one end and an inspiration valve at the other. This gradually assisted in the resolution of the two problems mentioned. Subsequently, the Volumatic (Allen and Hanbury) was developed and more recently the Rondo (Tillotts). All these devices have the disadvantage that they are very cumbersome and therefore are most useful for the administration of twice-daily prophylactics, in which case they can be left at home. The Nebuhaler and Volumatic can be taken apart and would fit into a handbag but not into the pocket of a pair of shorts.

The large expansion chambers do not demand hand–breath coordination. One or several puffs may be propelled into one of the larger devices and the patient can adopt a technique similar to that employed in the use of the solo metered-dose inhaler. However some people, particularly small children perhaps would find it easier to inhale from the device during normal tidal breathing with no breath-holding. This is less predictable but achieves results, especially if two or three breaths are used to flush out the device's chamber.

Unfortunately, the nozzles and canisters of metered-dose inhalers manufactured by different companies are not compatible, although there has been some agreement on the colour coding of devices (blue for a beta$_2$-agonist, brown for an inhaled steroid). The compatibility of different inhalers with the two principal expansion chambers, either using the whole of an original metered-dose inhaler or simply the canister, is shown in Table 7.1.

Table 7.1 Compatibility table of metered-dose aerosol inhalers and expansion chambers.

Trade names/Preparations	Nebuhaler	Volumatic
Ventolin (salbutamol)	X	✓
Becotide/Becloforte (beclomethasone)	X	✓
Bricanyl (terbutaline)	✓	X
Pulmicort (budesonide)	✓	X
Atrovent (ipratropium)	✓	✓
Intal (sodium cromoglycate)	✓	X
Tilade (nedocromil sodium)	✓	X
Berotec (fenoterol)	✓	✓
Bronchodil (reproterol)	X	✓
Ventide (salbutamol/beclomethasone)	X	✓

There is an adaptor to allow Intal and Tilade inhalers to be used with a Nebuhaler.
✓ – compatible; X – incompatible.

Dry powder devices

When it was first introduced, sodium cromoglycate (Intal) was available only in a dry powder preparation, the spincap, which was taken using a

Spinhaler. The device perforated the side of the capsule then relied upon a breath-operated propeller and centrifugal force to project the powder into the inhaled airstream. Whistles are available which encourage children to suck and not to blow. The original spincaps contained an inert carrier, lactose, but they now contain only 20 mg of micronized sodium cromoglycate. The original Spinhaler has evolved and the current device has a special flange to meet the lips, so that the mouthpiece passes between the teeth, to avoid impaction of the inhaled powder on the front of the teeth.

As the dry powder device requires no special co-ordination to operate it, just sufficient inspiration to draw the powder into the lungs, several companies have developed one. Salbutamol (Ventolin) is produced in rotacaps, which contain 200 or 400 μg of microfine salbutamol and a lactose carrier of larger size particle. Beclomethasone (Becotide) is also produced in a rotacap containing 100, 200 or 400 μg of the drug. Rotacaps are taken via a Rotahaler which, after breaking the capsule in half, uses a vortex effect to swirl the powder into the airstream. Usually it is possible to empty the capsule in one or two sucks starting from the end of a gentle expiration and holding the breath for 10 seconds afterwards.

Originally introduced as a substitute for those who could not use a pressurized aerosol, dry powder devices are now first choice for many asthmatics and would be even more popular if they were self-contained.

The Diskhaler, for salbutamol and beclomethasone (Ventodisks and Becodisks), is a flat device that takes a disc containing 8 metered doses of the drug in a small blister. The drug is microfine and accompanied by a lactose carrier—the carrier is slightly sweet and is designed to fall into the mouth while the active drug progresses down the airways. The inspiratory flow rate is less than for the Rotahaler. More recently, the Turbohaler was introduced for use with terbutaline (Bricanyl). This device is small and contains 200 doses of 0.5 mg dry powder terbutaline and no carrier. A similar device for use with budesonide (Pulmicort) is awaited.

Children are often confused about sucking and blowing. In order to explain the difference it is necessary to demonstrate it—blowing out candles and sucking a drink up a straw. A gadget called a Tri-flo is very useful in this respect. It has three tubes each attached together and to a tube which can be sucked. At the bottom of each tube is a different coloured plastic ball which is drawn to the top of the tube, depending on the force of the inspiration—more visual in the initial instruction process (Fig. 7.4).

Another practical problem with small children is that the novelty of an inhaler may soon wear off and parents will have to be patient and will also require sensitive support in their endeavours. Some children can use an aerosol-cum-expansion chamber at 2 years old, breath-operated dry powder devices by 3 years old and aerosol inhalers by 7 – 8 years old. A soft face mask has now been fitted to administer drugs via a Nebuhaler to enable either prophylactic drugs or ipratropium to be administered easily to small

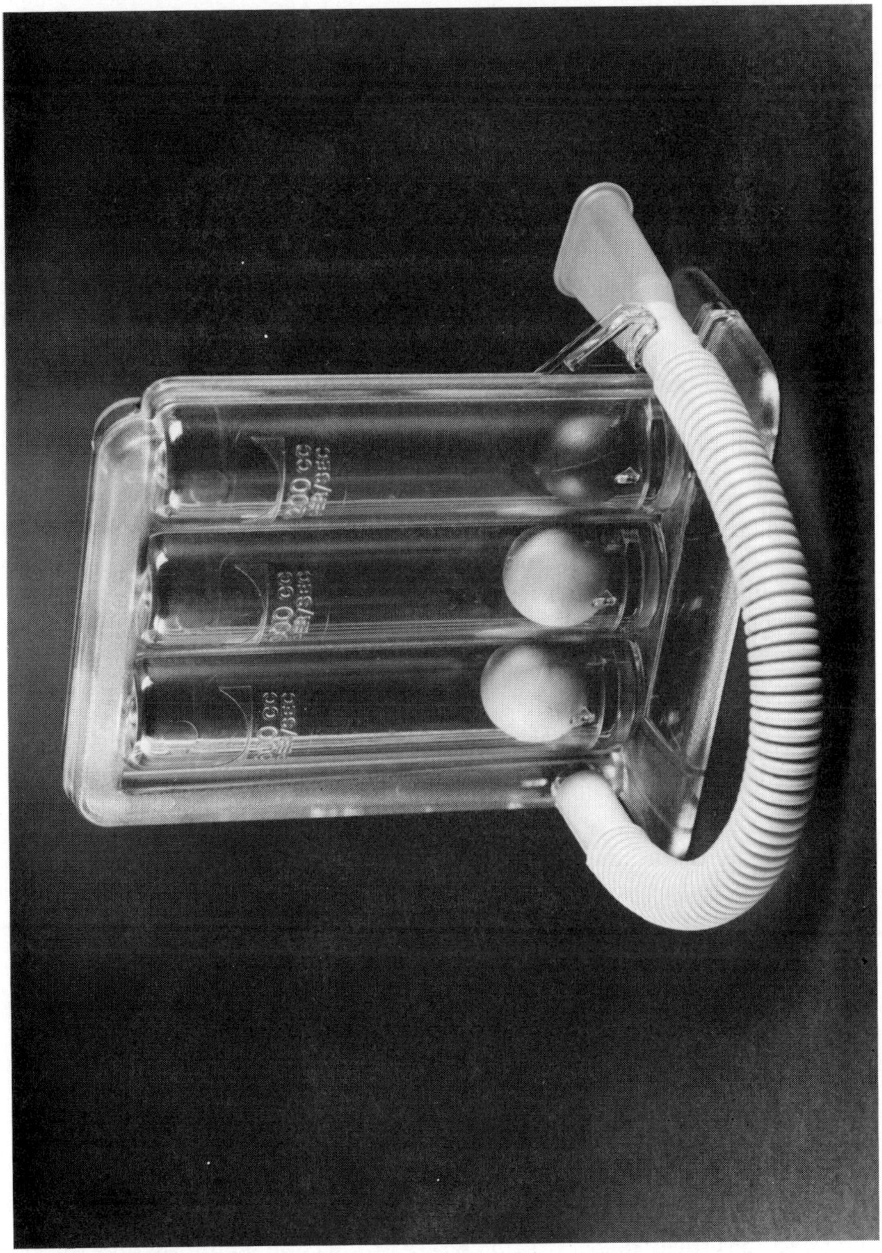

Figure 7.4 Tri-flo.

infants who are not yet capable of using a Nebuhaler in their mouths. The time taken is far shorter than using a nebulizer. But remember that a sizeable proportion of the population finds it impossible to use an aerosol inhaler whatever their age!

It is most important that the GP or nurse is thoroughly conversant with any devices that may have been prescribed for the patient. The working of these devices must be properly explained and demonstrated to the patient, and then the patient's technique must be sympathetically tested.

It is not appropriate here to provide detailed instructions on how to operate each device; this should be done actually using the particular device. With all low-dose inhaled preparations it is vital to pay close attention to detail in following the manufacturer's instructions on technique, for instance loading and preparing a dry powder device before inhalation. Two important points are that neither aerosol jets nor powder will pass through teeth, which should not obstruct passage of the drug, no devices benefit from having damp exhaled air breathed into them, especially dry powder devices.

Poor technique may lead to the loss of small but critical amounts of therapeutic agent. Always satisfy yourself that the patient understands and is competent to use the device prescribed.

Aerosol inhalers may become less widely used as the concern over the ozone layer and chlorofluorocarbon propellants grows, even though the volumes involved are relatively small. Set against this, many of the newer dry powder devices are considerably more expensive than their aerosol counterparts.

Nebulizers

Nebulized preparations are available for those patients who:

1 are too young to use other devices, but need inhaled therapy;
2 hopelessly co-ordinated but need inhaled therapy;
3 have a very low inspiratory volume;
4 need inhalation of a drug over a period of time.

A nebulizer is a device that produces a finely dispersed cloud of droplets containing the therapeutic agent. The droplets may be inhaled through a mask or a mouthpiece. Ideally, the droplets should be 2 – 5 μm in diameter for maximum penetration. Larger droplets are deposited before they reach the smaller airways, the desired sites of action. A flow rate of 6 – 8 litres/minute is desirable to achieve nebulization of 3 ml of solution within 10 minutes.

Jet nebulizers work on the same principle as a paint spray, i.e. by blowing air across the end of a pipe dipped below the fluid's surface: the aspirated fluid becomes finely dispersed, the larger droplets precipitating on a 'baffle' (Fig. 7.5).

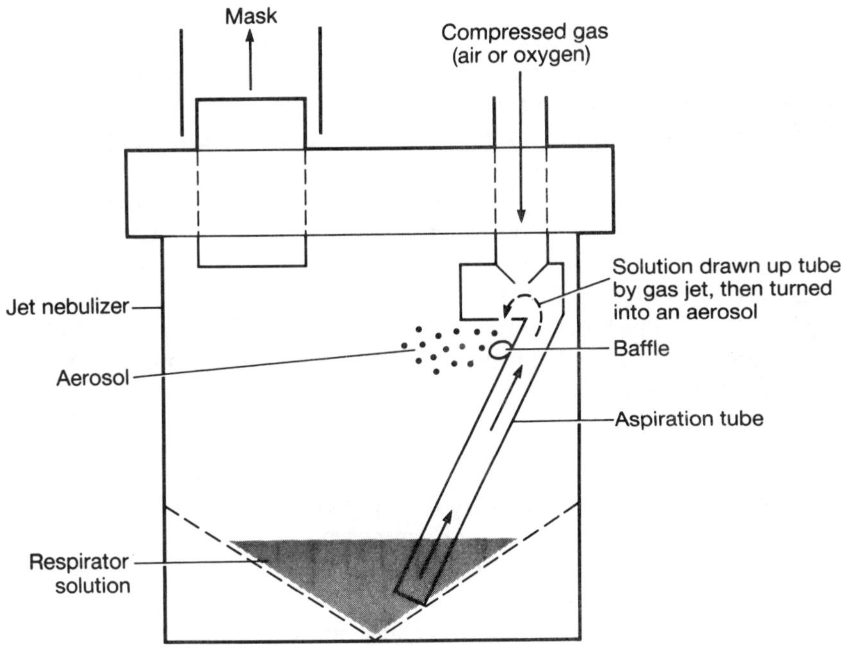

Figure 7.5 Jet nebulizer.

Jet nebulizers are usually used in conjunction with a portable air pump which provides filtered, oil-free air at the appropriate rate to obtain the correct particle size. Oxygen is often/usually used in hospital wards, sometimes because it is necessary and sometimes because it is the most convenient medium. Ultrasonic nebulizers are quiet and work via the vibration of fluid by a piezo-electric transducer at ultrasonic frequencies.

Although apparent dosages are large, only about 10% of this reaches the lungs, as in co-ordinated aerosol inspiration. With a nebulizer, much of the drug enters the ambient air and is wasted. In addition, there is always some fluid left in the bottom of the device which represents a large proportion of a small original volume.

Nebulizers can be used for the administration of salbutamol, terbutaline, fenoterol, reproterol, sodium cromoglycate, ipratropium bromide and even beclomethasone suspension.

Injection

Asthma drugs may be injected, usually in acute situations, but infusions may be required over a long period.

In the past, subcutaneous adrenaline and intravenous aminophylline were the most popular anti-asthma agents. Today subcutaneous, intramuscular or slow-intravenous selective beta$_2$-agonists are more likely to be used (*see* page 76 for dosage of salbutamol), but now that nebulized bronchodilators are freely and safely available such less used routes are not in widespread clinical use, although in the presence of severe obstruction, with mucus-plugging, the intravenous route may be more effective. In some patients with severe nocturnal symptoms, continuous subcutaneous injection of terbutaline has been used.

Intravenous aminophylline still has a role in two situations.

1 In acute cases, when a patient has failed to respond to beta$_2$-agonists and before corticosteroids have had any effect, aminophylline is given as a slow bolus injection over 15 minutes.
2 In the event of severe asthma failing to respond to adequate doses of conventional therapy—systemic corticosteroids, beta$_2$-agonists and possibly anticholinergics—an infusion of aminophylline for a protracted period may improve symptoms.

Great care must be taken when administering intravenous aminophylline, in case the patient has been taking long-acting oral theophylline preparations.

Hydrocortisone may be given by intravenous injection, in a dose of 100 – 500 mg, but usually only if the patient might vomit or is in respiratory failure.

8 The Management of Asthma and the Organization of Care

Current deficiencies – Overcome underdiagnosis – Patient's history is important – Examination – Flow chart of diagnosis and treatment – Occasional bronchoconstriction merits $beta_2$-agonist therapy – Bronchial hyperreactivity needs to be suppressed – Severe mucosal inflammation requires corticosteroid therapy – Urge regular prophylactic therapy – Relief of symptoms, preventive therapy and treatment of acute severe asthma in infancy and early childhood, later childhood, adolescence and adulthood – Minimum therapy for maximum effect – Treat severe asthma vigorously – ?Antibiotics – Beware the 'silent chest' – Hay fever – Eczema – Illustrative case histories

The Organization of Care

Anticipatory care – Use self referral to hospital only in special circumstances – Long term follow up – Patient's role is central – Patient self reliance – The nurse's role in asthma care? – Asthma diaries? – Asthma register – Care needs time – Written explanations and instructions for patient – Referral to hospital – Why? – When? – Admission of asthmatic patients should be to a thoracic medicine unit – Nurses need training – Need for audit

In planning future strategies in asthma care it is important to examine past and present deficiencies. The British Thoracic Association concluded after its study of mortality from asthma that the deficiencies were:

- underdiagnosis;
- inadequate use of prophylactic therapy;
- failure to recognize the severity of exacerbations;
- undertreatment of acute exacerbations;
- poor follow up;
- minimal patient education.

Although there have been tremendous advances in our understanding of asthma and its treatment, there has been a delay in passing the benefits of these advances on to our patients, often for the reasons outlined on the previous page. Although the situation is improving slowly, there can be no room for complacency. The aim of asthma therapy is to enable the patient to lead a normal life, which is best achieved by tailoring therapy to the needs of each individual patient within a structured framework. The vast majority of patients will conform to a predictable pattern, based upon the person, individual susceptibility, age, sex, history, symptoms and physical findings, including the results of lung function tests. We should aim to produce optimal results for the individual and not to settle for a mediocre value of function that, although conforming to a table of predicted values, may be far short of what is possible. The first priority is to make the diagnosis before progressively assessing the problem and matching the treatment to the problem.

Underdiagnosis

A staggering level of underdiagnosis appears to exist in some quarters. To remedy this it might be wise to 'screen' schoolchildren and introduce specific questions related to asthma into school medicals, together with the routine use of PEFR measurements. Most asthmatics consult their GPs about respiratory symptoms which appear to be related to viral respiratory tract infections. Sometimes this attribution is erroneous in that there is no true evidence of infection, and the wheeze and cough, which may in the past have been associated with, or triggered by, a respiratory tract infection, are simply symptoms of asthma. It is up to the GP to ask the right questions during history taking. The inquisitive, informed and articulate middle-class parent is far more likely to obtain a diagnosis of 'asthma' than a more retiring parent who will meekly accept another irrelevant and inappropriate antibiotic prescription for 'bronchitis'.

The definition of asthma must always be borne in mind, remembering that asthma is a disorder of function that may be precipitated by many different factors or may sometimes be without apparent cause. Symptoms (wheeze, cough and breathlessness) must be balanced against pathological features (bronchoconstriction, mucosal oedema and increased mucus secretion). It is not satisfactory to search for a wheeze. An attempt should be made to quantify the problem and measure a variable that depends on bronchial airflow, such as the PEFR.

Patients who consult their GP with respiratory problems should be approached with a high index of suspicion and GPs must be prepared to be honest with patients and parents. The level of underdiagnosis is strong evidence that asthma is not always an obvious diagnosis. Morever, it is a time-consuming diagnosis to make. However, the temptation to write a prescription for an antibiotic must be resisted, knowing that impatient patients are waiting to be seen. Although correct diagnosis and appropriate treatment may take more time, they should lead to better patient management, well-informed patients and greater professional satisfaction. The time taken to change ingrained patient attitudes regarding diagnosis and treatment may be considerable, but it is worthwhile.

There is a considerable overlap of symptom patterns irrespective of the patient's age, even though the differential diagnosis may change with age. When a patient presents for the third time in a year with a cough and wheeze, perhaps precipitated by a cold, further inquiry is necessary. It may be inappropriate, especially if the patient is unwell, to make an in-depth inquiry, but a few questions regarding exercise tolerance and nocturnal cough and wheeze between these exacerbations may indicate a working diagnosis of asthma. Diagnoses in isolation are valueless, other than for statistical purposes, but a diagnosis that leads to effective management and a satisfactory outcome is the very purpose of medicine.

It may be reasonable to inquire into a family history of asthma, atopy or 'bronchitis'. Always ascertain what these diagnostic labels mean to the patient, because their concept may be quite different from the GP's.

When a patient presents with a cough, wheeze and breathlesssness, it is important to consider the differential diagnosis (*see* pages 40 – 6). This process is easier in the young patient because the diagnostic possibilities are fewer, and ageing, coupled with smoking and environmental hazards, will often produce a complex cardiorespiratory problem. Nonetheless, a history will contribute greatly to the diagnostic process.

- Is there a cough?
- Is it productive?
- If so, what is the sputum like?
- When does it occur?
- What provokes it?
- Is there wheezing or noisy breathing?
- Is it worse at night?
- What happens at night if the patient wakes breathless?
- At what time does the patient awake breathless?
- Is there heartburn or acid reflux at night?
- Is there chest pain?
- Is the patient aware of a change in their heart beat?
- Does the patient smoke or has the patient smoked?
- If so, how much?
- Did the patient have similar symptoms in childhood?
- Is the patient on medication for this problem?

- Does it provide relief?
- Is the patient on medication for hypertension or angina (beta-blockers), arthritis (NSAIDs), glaucoma (beta-blocker eye drops)?
- Does the patient have hay fever?
- Does the patient wheeze as part of their hay fever?

Physical examination should start with general observation of the patient: colour (cyanosis or pallor), finger-clubbing, stained fingers from cigarette smoking, abnormal lymph glands, the position of the trachea, the presence of a goitre. Next, it is important to observe chest movements, examining the possible use of accessory muscles of respiration and chest symmetry. Palpation of the chest during inspiration and expiration may reveal palpable 'crackles' or the 'hardness' of severe asthma when there is marked obstruction to expiration. Percussion of the chest may reveal normal resonance or extension of resonance over the liver and, finally, auscultation should be performed to assess the breath sounds and to detect the presence of added sounds such as wheezes, which are polyphonic and diffuse in asthma, and inspiratory crackles and rattles, which may be localized or widespread.

The importance of the cardiovascular system will depend on age. The heart rate and rhythm should be monitored first, then the blood pressure, before examining the heart itself. It may be necessary to perform an ECG or a chest X-ray. In uncomplicated asthma a chest X-ray will contribute little. However, if the asthma is not straightforward a chest X-ray may reveal a collapsed lobe, especially the middle lobe of the right lung (Fig. 8.1), a pneumothorax, mediastinal emphysema (Fig. 8.2) or asthma that is more intense in one lung than in the other.

When the field of investigation has been narrowed down to the lungs, it is necessary, as well as performing an examination and perhaps X-ray, to have a structured approach to diagnosis, which may lead at the same time to a rational approach to therapy. When the asthma programme was developed in our practice, we explored a team approach that involved the practice's doctors and nurses. We felt that it was necessary to summarize our agreed policy in the form of a flow chart. This flow chart would work through diagnosis and assessment to therapy, with the emphasis on principles and not on degrees of urgency, which in the clinical situation would clearly also have a profound influence.

One of our basic tenets was to strip asthma of the veil of mystery with which some might try to enshroud it. We have seen that the pathological processes involved in asthma are highly complex but to obtain good results we have to reduce them to simple proportions and relate them to logical therapy. There are exceptions but most cases of asthma can be dealt with in this way. Good treatment demands patient participation; patients are not passive spectators and must be actively involved in their own treatment,

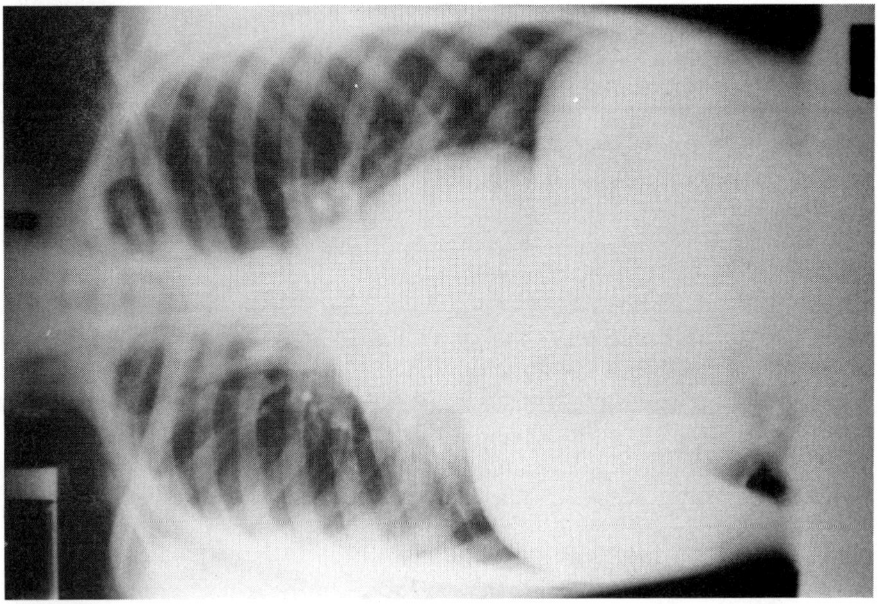

Figure 8.1(a) Collapse of middle lobe of right lung in exacerbation of asthma.

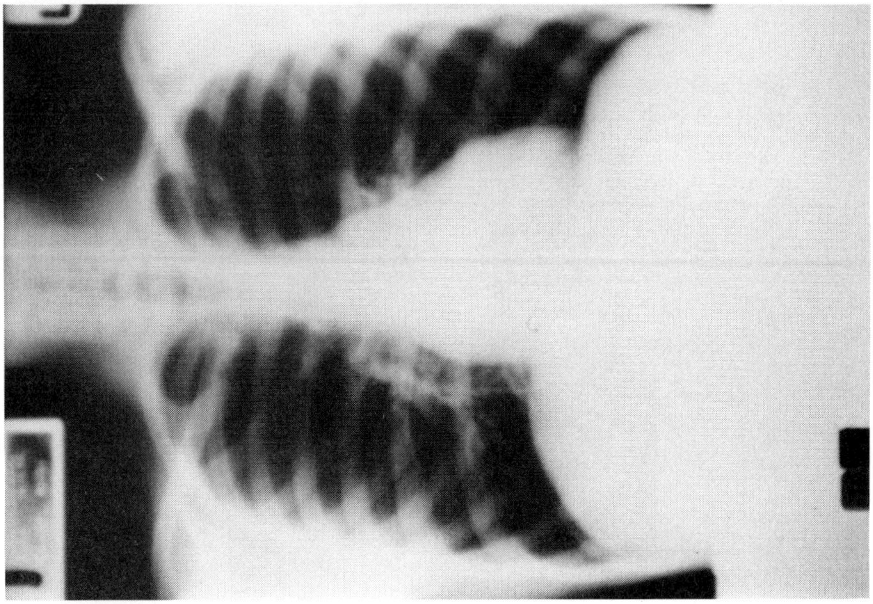

Figure 8.1(b) After re-expansion.

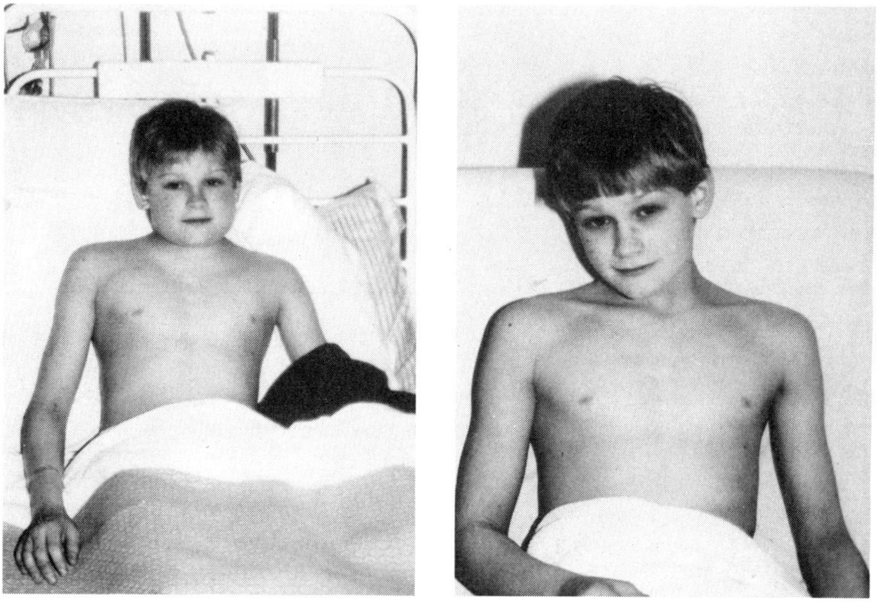

On presentation 2 weeks later

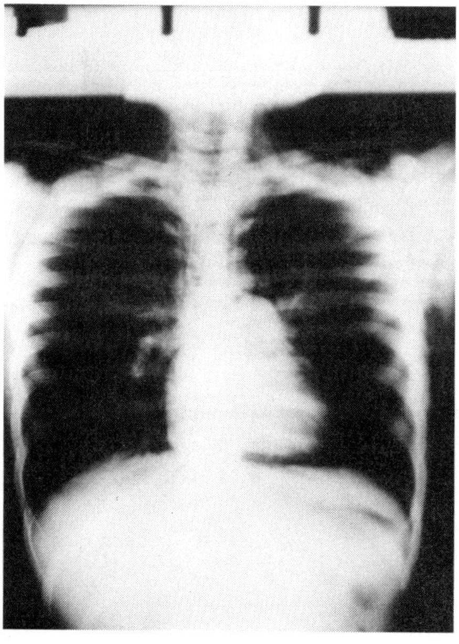

Figure 8.2 Mediastinal emphysema.

certainly in understanding it and its rationale. Attitudes are slow to change, but one of the most important factors in recent improvements in diabetic care has been the demystification of diabetes so that properly educated patients look after their own day-to-day management with advice and back up from their doctors.

The flow chart (Fig. 8.3, *see* pages 108 – 9) is based on principles and it would now be most sensible if we considered the diagnostic section alone.

Let us suppose that asthma is a strong possibility.

- Does this patient have asthma?
- Measure the PEFR or spirometry.

We may then take course I, in which the patient has no symptoms or signs at the time and has PEFR figures which are close to or above the predicted levels for that person.

- No airflow limitation at present time.
- Can asthma be provoked? (e.g. exercise test—page 71)
- Can asthma be confirmed? (history, home monitoring of PEFR)

If asthma is not confirmed, it is important to arrive at an alternative diagnosis and to keep an open mind for the future, as the diagnosis may have to be reconsidered depending on events. A positive exercise test, or home monitoring that confirms abnormal bronchial lability, will confirm a diagnosis of asthma; the ability to block or reverse the airflow limitation will add weight to the diagnosis.

Course II is followed if the patient has symptoms or signs suggestive of asthma, or has PEFR figures which are below 85% of the predicted value. Remember that apparently 'normal' values may occur in some symptomatic patients whose lung function tests would normally yield results up to 25 – 30% above average.

- Can the airflow limitation be reversed with an inhaled bronchodilator (either $beta_2$-agonist or anticholinergic)?
- A return to predicted or previous best values suggests bronchoconstriction.
- Values that are still much lower than predicted levels suggest mucosal inflammation, with mucosal oedema and mucus plugging, or a structural disorder.
- Combined use of regular bronchodilator therapy with a two week trial of systemic corticosteroids, such as prednisolone, should produce a marked improvement in the case of asthma and suggests the presence of a mucosal element.
- Absence of a measurable response suggests an irreversible structural abnormality.

Vigilance produces diagnoses.

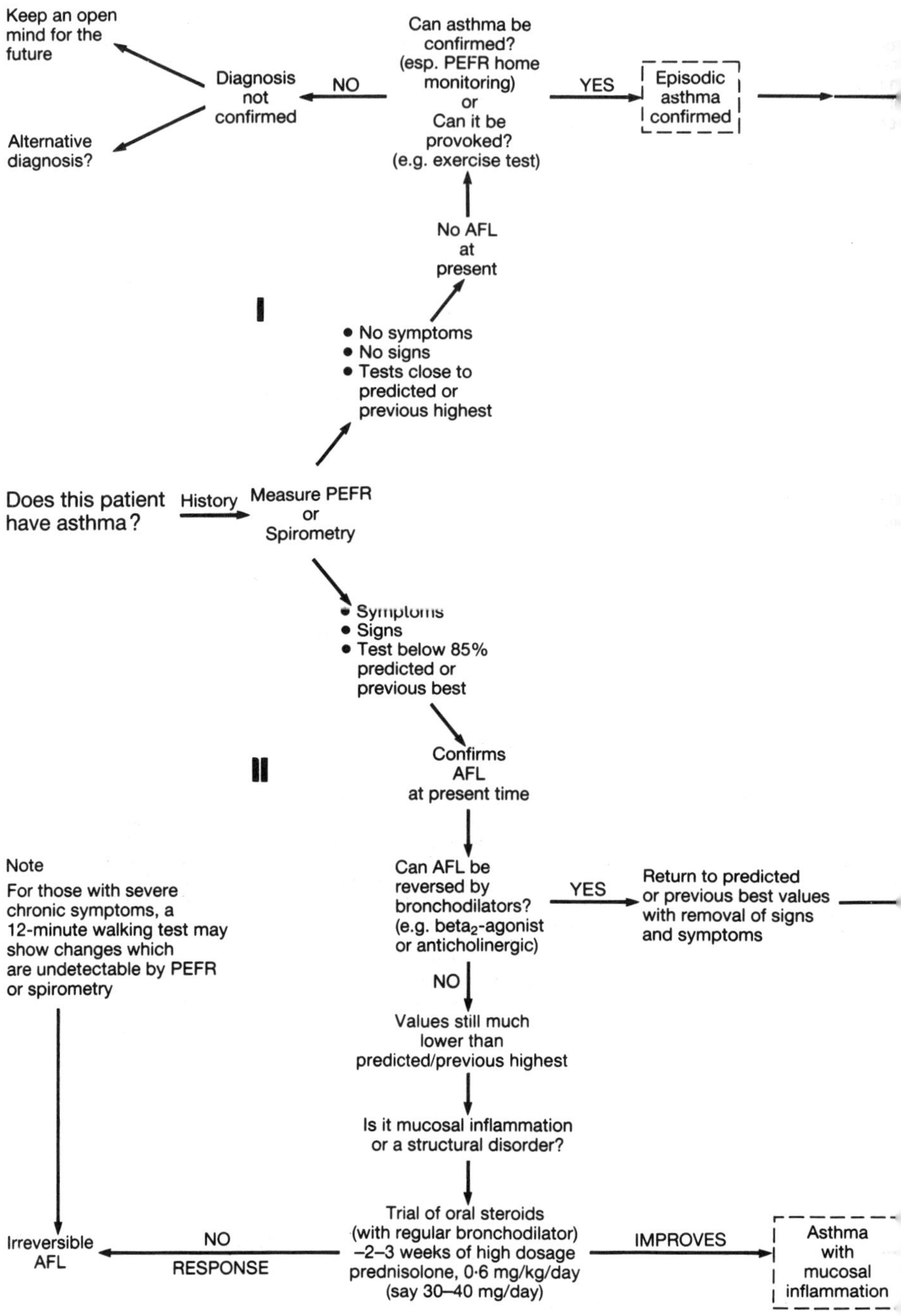

Figure 8.3 Diagnosis and management of asthma.

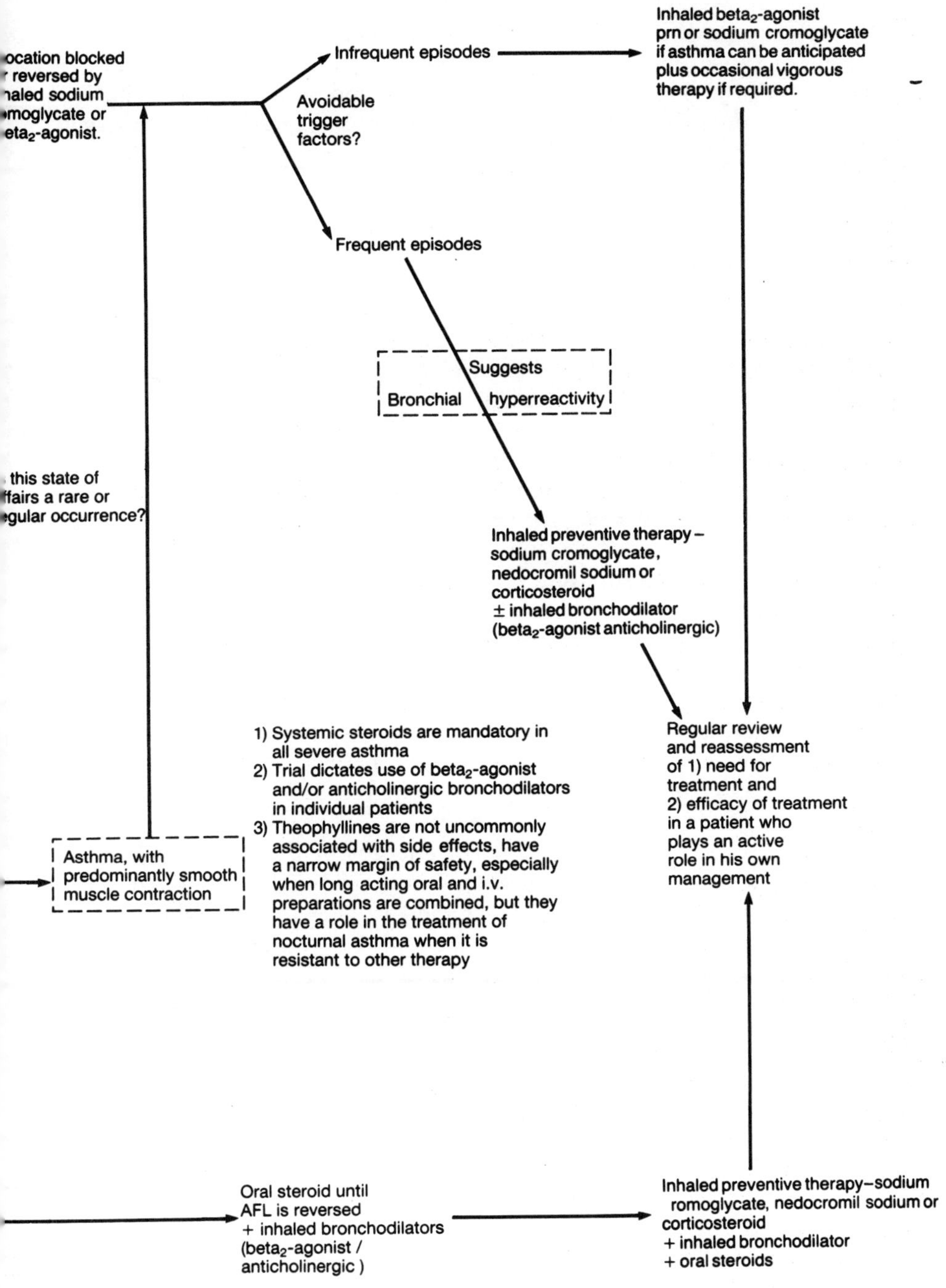
ocation blocked
r reversed by
haled sodium
moglycate or
eta2-agonist.
Infrequent episodes
Avoidable
trigger
factors?
Inhaled beta2-agonist
prn or sodium cromoglycate
if asthma can be anticipated
plus occasional vigorous
therapy if required.
Frequent episodes
Suggests
Bronchial hyperreactivity
this state of
ffairs a rare or
egular occurrence?
Inhaled preventive therapy –
sodium cromoglycate,
nedocromil sodium or
corticosteroid
± inhaled bronchodilator
(beta2-agonist anticholinergic)
Regular review
and reassessment
of 1) need for
treatment and
2) efficacy of treatment
in a patient who
plays an active
role in his own
management
1) Systemic steroids are mandatory in all severe asthma
2) Trial dictates use of beta2-agonist and/or anticholinergic bronchodilators in individual patients
3) Theophyllines are not uncommonly associated with side effects, have a narrow margin of safety, especially when long acting oral and i.v. preparations are combined, but they have a role in the treatment of nocturnal asthma when it is resistant to other therapy
Asthma, with
predominantly smooth
muscle contraction
Oral steroid until
AFL is reversed
+ inhaled bronchodilators
(beta2-agonist /
anticholinergic)
Inhaled preventive therapy–sodium
romoglycate, nedocromil sodium or
corticosteroid
+ inhaled bronchodilator
+ oral steroids

Although a case could be made for opportunistic measurement of PEFR with a brief enquiry about breathlessness or cough, full advantage should be taken of those opportunities that present, with the regular bouts of 'bronchitis', 'bronchial', or 'bronichal', often superimposed on a background of regular tolerated symptoms. We should not passively encourage middle-aged and newly retired non-smokers to accept increasing asthmatic symptoms as a part of the ageing process.

The principles of treatment

The purpose of this book is to present a relatively simple, logical approach to the treatment of asthma based on my own experience. If this approach is adopted, only a very small minority of asthma sufferers will have difficulty in managing their condition. Moreover, if followed, the principles of the approach outlined here will not lead to any detriment to the patient apart from the even smaller minority who have steroid-resistant asthma.

Before proceeding however, it must be noted that implicit in these principles is the overriding recognition that all severe asthma, whether of acute onset, insidiously subacute or chronic, demands the prompt use of adequate doses of corticosteroids. Also, while asthma tends to be predictable in the medium term, it can occasionally behave unpredictably and become acutely severe in the long term.

As patients are our professional raison d'etre they must be involved in their own treatment from the beginning. Prophylactic therapy relies upon a very high level of patient compliance, and a patient who does not grasp the importance of the therapy and its preventive role is unlikely to take it reliably.

Treatment must relate to our current concept of the pathophysiology of asthma and this is summarized simply in the flow chart and Fig. 8.4. Asthma, however, is a dynamic disorder and with time patients will transfer between groups. This change can often be observed during the course of a single year, for instance during the hay fever season.

The drugs used to treat asthma may be divided, in practical terms, into those that:

1 dilate the bronchi by relaxing the smooth muscle; or
2 modify the inflammatory process in the bronchial wall.

Clearly, the various components of the asthma process require different therapy (Fig. 8.4).

(a) Occasional fully reversible bronchoconstriction

Occasional fully reversible bronchoconstriction is most commonly treated with a bronchodilator, usually a beta$_2$-agonist such as salbutamol, as

PATHOPHYSIOLOGY	TREATMENT
(a) Occasional, fully reversible airflow limitation (bronchoconstriction)	Inhaled beta$_2$-agonist, as required
(b) Evidence of bronchial hyperreactivity (clinical symptoms and lability of PEFR) – i.e. inflammation, with reversible airflow limitation (bronchoconstriction)	*Add* inhaled sodium cromoglycate, nedocromil sodium or corticosteroids (if *very* unstable, oral corticosteroids)
(c) Evidence of severe mucosal inflammation (productive cough and airflow limitation refractory to inhaled beta$_2$-agonist – i.e. not bronchoconstriction alone)	*Add* oral (systemic) corticosteroids (introduce or revise dosage of inhaled prophylactic therapy)

Figure 8.4 Summary of the principles of treatment.

required. The route of administration will depend upon the patient's age, the disease's severity and individual factors, but for an occasional problem inhalation is the most immediate and effective route. If the bronchoconstriction is short lived, oral beta$_2$-agonists, oral theophyllines or inhaled ipratropium are not appropriate because of the delay in their onset of action.

Problems may arise over the definition of the word 'occasional'. If 'occasional' means several times a day or even several times a week, perhaps waking up in the night sometimes, the patient's condition falls under 'bronchial hyperreactivity' (*see* below). Concern over the unaccompanied use of increasing doses of inhaled beta$_2$-agonists is that they may contribute to the unstable behaviour of the bronchial smooth muscle, thereby increasing the swings in airflow limitation.

Although the distinction between occasional and more frequent occurrence of bronchoconstriction and the attendant use of inhaled beta$_2$-agonists may appear to be academic, it is not. To confirm the distinction, it may be instructive to ask the patient to record their PEFR at home to ascertain whether the background variability is within normal limits. If the asthma is truly occasional, the PEFR will fall within this range.

(b) Bronchial hyperreactivity

When there is evidence of bronchial hyperreactivity but the airflow limitation can be fully or effectively reversed, a different therapeutic approach is necessary. It is important to remember that many patients underestimate their symptoms or deliberately play them down so that they do not appear to be fussing unnecessarily. Therefore, it is essential to quantify the problem, through PEFR home monitoring, which will often demonstrate marked swings in the PEFR, with little provocation (Fig. 5.2, p. 59). Symptoms demanding relief with an inhaled beta$_2$-agonist are nocturnal asthma, a wheeze and a cough on rising and easily triggered asthma during the day, possibly on exercise or exposure to cigarette smoke, for example.

Bronchial hyperreactivity depends upon the effects of a low grade inflammatory reaction in the bronchial mucosa and submucosa. This bronchial hyperreactivity can persist for 3 – 4 weeks after a single exposure to an allergen for instance, even in the presence of relatively few inflammatory cells, such as eosinophils and mast cells.

Although it is difficult to avoid cold air, smoky or dusty environments and common cold viruses, it may be possible to take simple precautions such as regular vacuuming of bedrooms, damp wiping of smooth surfaces, and the avoidance of smoking, pets and drinks and food known to provoke asthmatic responses. However, there is a limit to the effectiveness of such measures even if the patient and his or her family become very obsessional about it.

The inflammatory reactions can be modified by several drugs which may be taken as inhaled prophylactic agents, e.g. sodium cromoglycate, nedocromil sodium and inhaled corticosteroids. These drugs are all distinct in their pharmacological properties, modes of action and the clinical situations to which they are best suited. They all have effects on the production or release of mediators and chemotactic factors, which either cause the asthmatic process directly or attract other cells that produce further mediators.

Prophylactic agents need to be taken regularly in order to maintain suppression of the inflammatory process. If they are not, a state of instability returns, which leads to increasing beta$_2$-agonist consumption. This is a common problem. Unfortunately, because the patient finds relief on most occasions from the beta$_2$-agonist, it is taken more often, while the prophylactic agent is rejected and discontinued as being of no value. This situation underlines the important role of patient education. There is no point in prescribing a drug whose action leads to no immediate result without explaining this to the patient. The possible roles of these prophylactic agents are discussed more fully in the sections devoted to the effect of age in selecting therapeutic agents and their means of administration (p. 115).

Another problem is when to stop a trial of therapy if it is not proving effective. I consider that when a patient is known to have unstable asthma the uncomfortable, distressing and dangerous symptoms should be treated as soon as possible. Unless the symptoms are very mild and the swings are small, I would allow a maximum of 7 days, depending upon circumstances. Occasionally, when the swings in PEFR are thought to be dangerous, it may be necessary to adopt an approach as outlined in the category (c) below.

Doctors and patients often forget that the most effective way to avoid nocturnal asthma is to take appropriate prophylaxis during the day. If inflammation is suppressed during the day, a large element of nocturnal asthma will be controlled. It is much safer and simpler to do this than to have the added confusion of taking unnecessary theophylline at bedtime.

When asthma is stably controlled, something may slightly upset the equilibrium and provoke renewed symptoms and swings in the PEFR. If these oscillations are around the normal PEFR level, it may be necessary only to increase the level of prophylaxis to improve the situation and review it later.

An asthma audit within my own practice disclosed some interesting figures on the use of inhaled prophylactic agents in male patients in 1988 (Fig. 8.5). There was a higher proportion of patients on regular prophylaxis in the very young and adult age groups compared with older children and adolescents. This finding is compatible with the observation that asthma is generally less troublesome during adolescence.

(c) Evidence of severe mucosal inflammation

This evidence is manifest as airflow limitation resistant to bronchodilator therapy, usually accompanied by a cough that becomes productive. The

(a) Numbers of identified male asthmatics and the proportion receiving treatment in the 12 months to March 1988

Age	0–6 yrs	7–14 yrs	14–21 yrs	Over 21
Total number	23	70	48	192
% on *no* treatment	21%	24%	35%	32%
% on treatment	79%	76%	65%	68%

(b) Types of treatrnent received during 12 months to March 1988

Age	0–6 yrs	7–14 yrs	14–21 yrs	Over 21
Number on treatment	18	52	29	129
P.R.N. $beta_2$-agonist %	17%	31%	54%	18%
Regular $beta_2$-agonist %	83%	69%	46%	82%
Inhaled prophylactic %	72%	54%	59%	72%

Figure 8.5 Numbers of identified male asthmatics and the proportion receiving treatment in the 12 months to March 1988.

additional airway obstruction demands higher doses of inhaled bronchodilators such as those administered by nebulizer. However, larger amounts of low-dose inhaled prophylactic agents are ineffective because they are incapable of significantly reducing the aggressive inflammatory reaction, even if they could penetrate to the inflamed bronchi and bronchioles. The only effective therapy is a systemic corticosteroid, in adequate dosage for a sufficient length of time. It is necessary to continue with this therapy until the inflammation is suppressed, as witnessed by the absence of symptoms (cough, breathlessness) and signs (wheeze or crackles) and the return of PEFR values or spirometry measurements to normal or previous best values. Often, the last pathological feature to disappear is the low morning PEFR, which accompanies the cough and breathlessness experienced on rising.

It is easy to decide to prescribe systemic corticosteroids in the presence of an acute exacerbation. However, it is equally important to recognize the need for positive intervention during insidious deterioration which takes place over days or weeks, perhaps accelerated by upper respiratory tract infections. In this situation there is a slow increase in symptoms and physical limitation, reflected in a parallel fall in the PEFR. The patient becomes progressively more at risk as the mucosal inflammation and oedema increase. A sharp superimposed bronchoconstriction may have very serious, even fatal, consequences. During recovery, such patients may exhibit great instability of PEFR and be at increased risk of dying. An inadequate course of corticosteroids will not suppress the bronchial wall inflammation which will recur if the patient tries to rely solely on inhaled prophyiactic agents.

Nebulized corticosteroids should *not* be administered to patients suffering from a severe exacerbation of asthma. The doses involved are trifling and should not be looked upon as magical because they are delivered by a nebulizer.

If patients are known to run a predictable course in certain situations, it is sensible for those patients to have a reserve of prednisolone tablets at home and to take them when a certain situation arises which should be determined for each patient. Delaying by only 12 hours may allow a severe exacerbation to occur which could have been prevented. Examples of appropriate situations are subjectively increased dyspnoea which is unresponsive, or considerably less responsive and for a shorter period of time, to the usual dose of inhaled bronchodilator, or a fall in PEFR to a pre-set level without a return to normal after bronchodilator therapy. Action should be taken before a fall to 50% of normal levels has occurred, but that degree of drop, which persists after inhalation of a bronchodilator, is justification in itself.

After the patient's airways have returned to normal, it is important to reassess their clinical situation, to judge whether this event was very exceptional or due to inadequate prophylactic therapy. It is of paramount importance to enquire diligently how many prophylactic doses the patient forgets in an average week. We should not castigate patients, but a reinforcing plea and an explanation will suffice on most occasions. Explain to patients that a small loss of a tiny dose can have serious consequences and, if currently prescribed therapy is not taken in adequate dosage, additional agents, such as a theophylline, or maintenance systemic steroids, will not be effective. The central theme is that the patient and medical team work together: the patient informs the doctor of events and the patient should always be seen by the doctor when required.

Rational care must always have guidelines, but doctors and patients need to be adaptable with respect to medication and its administration. Both the drugs used and their means of administration will vary according to the age of the patient. For each age group, treatment will be considered in relation to the clinical picture and dealt with under two headings:

1 basic relief of symptoms and preventive therapy;
2 acute severe asthma.

Guidelines for all ages are summarized in (Fig. 8.6a and b).

Treatment

Treatment of asthma in infancy and early childhood

Many GPs find asthma in early childhood perplexing because it is difficult to assess and to treat. Asthma exemplifies the rule learnt from triage that those patients who make the most noise are usually not the ones who are most ill. Similarly, in infancy, there is a group of babies who have a distinct wheeze in the daytime, but who are rarely troubled by nocturnal symptoms. They are not distressed by their symptoms, nor is there any evidence of respiratory distress, such as a raised respiratory rate or an increased heart rate. However, the baby's parents may be very concerned and it is important to review the history and clinical findings with them, being prepared to reassess the baby if there is any change in the pattern of symptoms.

In contrast some infants are troubled by a regular night-time cough, which is usually disruptive enough to wake the parents and even the child, with wheezing and breathlessness often present. These children are clearly asthmatic; they will have acute exacerbations with viral respiratory tract infections. They experience breathlessness, a wheeze and a cough which is usually productive, suggesting significant mucosal involvment. This may also occur in some children who are otherwise asymptomatic. Exercise-induced symptoms are not a serious problem in the infant or toddler; they become important as the child gets older and becomes more active.

Category of asthma / Age	1–2 years	2–12 years	Above 12 years and atopic adults with 'mild' or seasonal asthma	Adults with persistent atopic and late-onset asthma
Occasional reversible A.F.L.	Inhaled ipratropium; after 15–18 months try inhaled beta$_2$-agonists (perhaps syrup before)	Inhaled beta$_2$-agonist as required	Inhaled beta$_2$-agonist, as required	NOT APPLICABLE
Recurrent reversible A.F.L. (bronchial hyperreactivity')	Inhaled bronchodilator + inhaled sodium cromoglycate ↓ inhaled corticosteroid if sodium cromoglycate inadequate	Inhaled beta$_2$-agonist + inhaled sodium cromoglycate ↓ inhaled corticosteroid if sodium cromoglycate inadequate (± theophylline at night)	Inhaled beta$_2$-agonist + inhaled sodium cromoglycate ↙ ↘ nedocromil sodium ⟷ corticosteroid if sodium cromoglycate inadequate (± theophylline at night)	Inhaled bronchodilator (beta$_2$-agonist or ipratropium) + nedocromil sodium or inhaled corticosteroid (± theophylline at night)
Persistent A.F.L. (more severe mucosal inflammation)	Inhaled bronchodilator + oral, soluble prednisolone (uncommon at this age) ↓ maintenance with sodium cromoglycate or inhaled corticosteroids	Inhaled beta$_2$-agonist + oral prednisolone until stable ↓ inhaled maintenance with sodium cromoglycate ↓ corticosteroids if sodium cromoglycate inadequate (± theophylline esp. at night)	Inhaled beta$_2$-agonist + oral prednisolone until stable ↓ maintain on inhaled sodium cromoglycate ↙ ↘ nedocromil sodium ⟷ inhaled corticosteroid if sodium cromoglycate inadequate (± theophylline at night)	Inhaled bronchodilator (beta$_2$-agonist/ipratropium) + oral prednisolone until stable ↙ ↘ nedocromil sodium ⟷ inhaled corticosteroid (± theophylline, esp. at night) (± maintenance steroids)

Figure 8.6 (a)

Means of Administration / Age	1–2 years	2–4 years	4–8 year	>8 years and adults
Oral	✓ Bronchodilator syrup + exceptional soluble prednisolone	(✓) Not first choice except 1) oral prednisolone 2) oral theophylline	(✓) Not first choice, except 1) oral prednisolone 2) oral theophylline	(✓) Not first choice, except 1) oral prednisolone 2) oral theophylline 3) in elderly
Nebulizer	? Best avoided below about 18 months as its use may worsen the asthma	(✓) Not ideal, because of time-factor in regular treatment - e.g. bronchodilator sodium cromoglycate or beclomethasone, but good for bronchodilator in exacerbations	(✓) Not usually appropriate for regular therapy but good for bronchodilator in exacerbations	(✓) Only appropriate in adults with high dosage - demand for bronchodilator, otherwise good for bronchodilators in exacerbations
M.D.I. + large volume spacer ± mask	(✓) May be used for ipratropium treatment below 18 months, also good for preventive therapy, e.g. sodium cromoglycate/corticosteroids	✓ May be used for bronchodilator but especially good for preventive therapy e.g. sodium cromoglycate/corticosteroids	✓ Rarely used for bronchodilator except in exacerbations, especially good for inhaled preventive therapy sodium cromoglycate/steroids	✓ Especially good for inhaled corticosteroids for good, even bronchial distribution - also for sodium cromoglycate + nedocromil sodium
M.D.I. (metered dose inhaler)	○ Not appropriate	○ Not appropriate	○ (✓) Occasional children are sufficiently well-co-ordinated	✓ A very convenient means of drug delivery if there is good hand/breath co-ordination
Dry powder devices	○ Not appropriate	○ (✓) A small proportion can master the technique	✓ Most convenient presentation especially good for bronchodilator in this age group + sodium cromoglycate and beclomethasone	✓ Effective means of drug presentation especially for the 30 per cent or so, who cannot used an M.D.I.

○ Never ? Perhaps (✓) Sometimes after due consideration ✓ Commonly

Figure 8.6 (b)

Basic relief of symptoms and preventive therapy

There are two principal problems in relieving symptoms in this age group: drugs and their administration.

$Beta_2$-agonists have no bronchodilator effect in patients under 15 – 18 months, although after this age they become progressively more effective. However, an unpredictable 40% of children in this age group will respond to inhaled ipratropium (the pathophysiology of asthma may be different in this 40% compared with the remaining 60%).

Administration presents difficulties, because changes in the osmolarity of the solution can cause bronchoconstriction during nebulized therapy. This bronchoconstriction cannot be relieved in those infants who do not respond to either the $beta_2$-agonists or the ipratropium being administered. Thus, the safety of nebulizer therapy in those infants under 18 months is in doubt. This bronchoconstriction does not occur when the same agents are administered from a metered-dose aerosol inhaler via a Nebuhaler, which can be fitted with a soft face mask to avoid the need to seal the lips around the Nebuhaler mouthpiece. However the drugs are administered, the child needs to be reasonably co-operative.

In the difficult age group of asthmatics of around 15 months, it may be justifiable to use a $beta_2$-agonist syrup, for example salbutamol diluted to 1 mg in 5 ml every 4 – 6 hours. It may bring some relief and it will not exacerbate the asthma.

Apart from nebulizer-induced bronchoconstriction, the Nebuhaler mask technique saves time each day. In infants under 18 months ipratropium can be tried, using 2 – 5 puffs into the Nebuhaler, but allowing two tidal breaths to clear the chamber before the next puff is triggered. Relief will be apparent after 30 minutes and this dosage can be repeated every 6 – 8 hours.

In the transitional age group where $beta_2$-agonists are becoming more effective, occasional symptoms may be treated with either the Nebuhaler (± face mask) with terbutaline (2 puffs, 500 μg) or the Volumatic with salbutamol (2 puffs, 200 μg). Exceptionally a nebulizer may be used with salbutamol respirator solution, for example, diluted down with physiological saline or in ready-to-use Nebules of 2.5 mg. Dosage may be repeated every 6 hours, if required.

The larger expansion chamber devices can be used with most co-operative children between the ages of 2 and 4 years, provided they have been adequately instructed in their use. By the age of about 4 years, dry powder devices such as the Rotahaler may be used to administer salbutamol, in a dosage of 200 – 400 μg, as needed or before exercise. Small children are able to use an expansion device with tidal breathing such as a Tri-flo, but the sucking action of other devices needs special instruction.

The more convenient a device is to use then the more likely it is to be used. Treatment must be seen to be in proportion to the problem.

Assessment must be clinical and based upon symptom patterns and physical signs. PEFR measurements can be inconsistent in patients under 4 years of age—some children under 4 years will be able to grasp the technique whereas some older children will find it difficult. Recurrent symptoms, nocturnal disturbances and a productive cough all indicate the need for additional suppressive therapy. The same age considerations are applicable when considering administration.

If there is evidence of frequent symptoms with cough and wheeze (whether by night or day), when the child is active and bronchodilators temporarily get rid of the symptoms and signs, sodium cromoglycate should be considered. Under 2 years of age, it can be given by nebulizer (20 mg in 2 ml) but, like all preparations given at this age, it might precipitate bronchoconstriction which must wear off spontaneously. As soon as the child is able to use it, a Nebuhaler and a sodium cromoglycate metered dose inhaler can be tried with 2 puffs (10 mg) 4 times daily, reducing to 1 puff 4 times daily if this provides adequate control. In the absence of a productive cough, a progressive response becomes apparent from between 1 and 6 weeks in the 65% of child asthmatics who respond to sodium cromoglycate. It should be borne in mind that symptoms continue to improve over several weeks. If symptoms have worsened in that time, or there has been no positive response, or the severity was underestimated originally, then I would institute therapy with an inhaled steroid such as budesonide, through a Nebuhaler (1 – 2 puffs of the low strength preparation, 50 – 100 μg, twice daily) or beclomethasone dipropionate via a Volumatic (2 puffs, 100 μg) which can be increased after about 4 days if control is inadequate. At this age, it would be unusual to require a daily dose of more than 400 μg of beclomethasone.

If there is a productive cough, even in the absence of severe asthma as judged by other criteria, this is indicative of more aggressive mucosal inflammation and warrants the use of a short course of soluble prednisolone (1 mg/kg body-weight/day). This achieves two results: rapid suppression of the very active inflammatory process and the reduction of mucus secretion to normal levels. The latter allows the low dose prophylactic agents to reach their target in the smaller bronchi and bronchioles and to maintain suppression of the inflammatory process. It is much too slow and less effective to treat well established asthma with low dose inhaled preventive therapy, especially if the bronchi are plugged, thereby preventing the even penetration of the low dose prophylactic agents.

Experience would suggest that the more severe the asthma and the younger it starts, the more likely it is to require inhaled corticosteroid therapy to keep it suppressed. However, as the safety profile of sodium cromoglycate is so good, it warrants a trial as the drug of choice in this age group. In the very small percentage of asthmatics who require inhaled steroids at this age but who cannot use an adaptation of the Nebuhaler, I have had success with nebulized beclomethasone dipropionate, even though the preparation is not ideal—2 ml (100 μg) of beclomethasone dipropionate suspension twice daily is usually sufficient.

In this age group, those children with productive coughs or whose asthma is exacerbated or precipitated by viral respiratory infections are more likely to require inhaled steroids as a prophylactic; presumably this reflects the mechanisms involved.

Oral theophyllines may be used, either as a syrup given every 6 hours or as a long acting preparation given once or twice daily (*see* page 87). However, great care must be taken to avoid dosages that result in toxic side effects, and it may be necessary to monitor blood levels. As theophyllines are usually administered orally, they need to be given in anticipation or as a form of prophylactic. I prefer to use inhaled bronchodilators (occasionally a beta$_2$-agonist syrup) and inhaled preventive agents (such as sodium cromoglycate and beclomethasone dipropionate) and save theophyllines for the rare occasions on which beta$_2$-agonists and preventive agents are insufficient.

Regardless of age, antibiotic therapy should be reserved for those occasions when there is good reason to believe that a susceptible bacterial infection is present, either on clinical grounds with a fever and later productive cough or by sputum examination for pathogenic organisms.

Acute severe asthma

Whatever the child's age, the parents need to remain quietly vigilant. If there is a change in the symptom pattern or a return of symptoms in those on preventive therapy, a closer watch needs to be maintained. Cough, breathlessness and wheeze may each be prominent to a varying degree and they respond only partially to the administration of bronchodilators. Except on the first such occasion, exacerbations of asthma will tend to run a similar course in any one patient. In such cases, if there is no productive cough it may be sufficient to double the dosage of inhaled preventive therapy until symptoms have gone and the asthmatic process has been suppressed. If this stage has passed and there is a productive cough and increasing bronchial airflow limitation, the administration of soluble prednisolone (Prednesol) is indicated, in a dosage of 1 – 2 mg/kg bodyweight/day, up to 20 mg. Inhaled beta$_2$-agonist and ipratropium should continue every 4 – 6 hours via a Nebuhaler (± mask) or nebulizer, depending upon the patient's age and level of co-operation. There is no evidence that corticosteroids are effective in the first year of life.

The assessment of severity is necessary in order to plan treatment and to decide whether hospital admission is necessary. The need for hospital admission will depend on several factors, some clinical and some environmental which should be taken into consideration irrespective of the patient's age.

- Breathlessness.
- Tight productive cough.
- Wheeze—presence or absence (beware the 'silent chest').
- Increasing respiratory rate (above 30 – 40 breaths/minute).
- Increasing heart rate (above 110 – 120 beats/minute).
- Restlessness.
- Inability to lie down or go to sleep.
- Use of accessory muscles of respiration.
- Intercostal/subcostal recession.
- Difficulty in eating, drinking and taking feeds.
- Difficulty in speaking more than staccato words.
- Cyanosis.
- Exhaustion.
- Distance from hospital.
- Quality of home care—competence and confidence of family.

If there is any doubt, it is safer to admit a patient to hospital than to persevere for too long at home. Inhaled bronchodilators may cause a ventilation/perfusion mismatch through patchy bronchodilatation which can lead to increased hypoxaemia. For this reason, it may be safer to drive the nebulizer with oxygen (at a flow rate of 6 – 8 litres/minute) rather than relying upon air from an electrical compressor.

If it is decided that rather than commencing therapy while the child's admission to hospital is arranged, it is clinically appropriate to treat the child at home, a repeated review of the clinical situation is necessary. Clinical review should cover two separate responses: namely, that to the inhaled bronchodilator and that to the systemic corticosteroids. (*NB* Their time courses are different; for example the response to prednisolone is much slower—there may be a feeling of improvement before any significant measureable change in spirometry or PEFR.) It is essential that the child's parents are in agreement with the decision to treat the child at home. The parents must be capable of acting as an extension of the doctor's eyes and hands. They must be competent and instructed in the danger signs to look out for.

As the smooth muscle component improves, the interval between the bronchodilator therapy can gradually be extended to 6 hours, and the dosage can be reduced as the asthma stabilizes. Prednisolone dosage should be maintained until the airways function has returned to normal. After this, the reduction in steroid dosage will depend upon three factors.

1 If the exacerbation has been truly acute then the prednisolone can be stopped abruptly after a return to normal, providing that therapy is for less than 2 weeks.
2 If the duration of the corticosteroid treatment is more than 2 weeks, there may be adrenocortical suppression and reduction should be graded, say 5 mg each day.
3 If the severe asthma was the culmination of a chronic picture of deterioration then the reduction in prednisolone dosage will need to be gradual, perhaps over several weeks, so that an incompletely suppressed inflammatory process does not flare up. While these adjustments to therapy are being made, prophylactic therapy should be considered or its dosage reviewed.

In summary:

Acute severe asthma

Inhaled bronchodilator:

Terbutaline— < 18 months say 5 puffs (1.25 mg) via Nebuhaler over 15 minutes, >18 months 0.2 ml (2 mg) of respirator solution, diluted to 2 ml in normal saline via nebulizer every 2 – 6 hours.

Salbutamol— >18 months say 2.5 mg in Nebule (2.5 ml) or by dilution of respirator solution, via nebulizer.

Ipratropium—<18 months 2 – 5 puffs (36 – 90 μg) via Nebuhaler, or >18 months 100 μg (0.4 ml nebulizer solution diluted to 2.5 ml in normal saline) via nebulizer

Systemic corticosteroids:

Prednesol— 1 – 2 mg/kg/day in a once daily oral dosage, up to 20 mg/day.

Hydrocortisone sodium succinate—100 mg i.v. if child is very ill and/or vomiting.

Preventive therapy:

Sodium cromoglycate—1 – 2 puffs (5 – 10 mg) 4 times daily via Nebuhaler, or (>18 months) 20 mg in 2 ml nebulizer solution, or 20 mg Spincap 4 times daily.

Beclomethasone—2 – 4 puffs (100 – 200 μg) via Volumatic, twice daily.

Budesonide— 1 – 2 puffs (50 – 100 μg) via Nebuhaler (± mask) twice daily.

Treatment of asthma in later childhood and adolescence

During childhood there are many changes in the clinical picture of asthma. By the age of 4 years, many children can be transferred from a large spacer device or a nebulizer to a dry powder inhaler for drug administration; by the age of 8 years, co-ordination will have improved further so that many children are able to use a metered dose inhaler on its own. At the age of about 8 years, many children can make a very positive contribution to their own management. However, in some children adolescence may herald an era of rebellion in which the treatment of their asthma may play a central role.

The natural history of asthma changes with the child's interaction with his or her environment. This is generally associated with increased activity. Allergy plays an increasing role in the mechanism of asthma, together with exercise-induced asthma and regular exposure to viral respiratory infections. With the child's increasing co-ordination and co-operation, it is possible to measure parameters of airways function, such as the PEFR, which contributes greatly to day-to-day monitoring and the assessment of any deterioration in function due to asthma.

Growth rate varies with age, but it may reflect good or inadequate control of the asthma or the overuse of corticosteroids to suppress symptoms. A typical clinical picture may include everything from mild, occasional, exercise symptoms through exacerbations related to viral infections, to regular nocturnal symptoms with cough and wheeze.

The choice of inhaler method should not depend solely on patient preference or the patient's ability to use a given inhaler (although these are very important considerations). The rule that the minimum effective dose should be used should always be borne in mind. With beta$_2$-agonists, tremor is the single most important side effect, especially with increasing age. However, bronchodilators need to be in a convenient form as they are likely to be carried about and a large spacer device would be quite impractical. Thus, metered dose inhalers or dry powder devices are interchangeable, depending upon the patient's ability. The possibility that inhaled corticosteroids may affect growth must not be overlooked and the use of an expansion chamber device will allow smaller doses to be used which are beneficial in the long run. Oropharyngeal thrush is more likely to occur in sensitive individuals with the use of inhaled corticosteroids taken as dry powder or by a metered dose aerosol inhaler when used alone. With twice daily administration of preventive agents every consideration should be given to the use of large spacer devices, such as the Nebuhaler or Volumatic, which allow a higher proportion of the inhaled dose to be spread evenly throughout the lungs. Metered dose inhalers on dry powder devices, which are more convenient to carry and to use, might be better suited for use with frequent administration, much as with sodium cromoglycate or nedocromil sodium, if higher doses of the latter are employed. Consistency of approach, in terms of minimizing the number of different inhalation devices, is another important consideration in the overall balance.

Basic relief of symptoms and preventive therapy

Simple bronchoconstriction will respond consistently to beta$_2$-agonist therapy. When there are occasional symptoms with an otherwise stable PEFR, a beta$_2$-agonist can be used in isolation. In the younger age group, a dry powder device, such as a Rotahaler, Diskhaler or Turbohaler, would be most appropriate. The Rotahaler and Diskhaler use salbutamol in a dosage of 200 or 400 μg and the Turbohaler uses terbutaline in a dosage of 500 μg. After the age of about 8 years, the child might wish to use a metered dose inhaler, but this should be allowed only if they are competent and consistent in technique.

Beta$_2$-agonists are very safe, but the need for a regular six-hourly regimen should suggest background bronchial hyperreactivity. Other indicators are nocturnal symptoms or excessive variations in PEFR measurements during home monitoring. Bronchial hyperreactivity, as a product of bronchial 'inflammation', demands the use of an inhaled anti-inflammatory preventive agent.

Most young asthmatics are atopic and sodium cromoglycate is still the prophylactic agent of first choice in this group. It needs to be administered 4 or more times daily and in the young child a Spinhaler, using Spincaps, is the most simple device, and contains 20 mg of sodium cromoglycate. Some children may find the inhaler form more acceptable. This can either be used alone or in the young via a Nebuhaler, in a dosage of 1 – 2 puffs (5 – 10 mg) 4 times daily. As in infancy and early childhood, this regimen, in conjunction with an inhaled beta$_2$-agonist, will lead to a progressive suppression of bronchial hyperreactivity in anything from 1 to 6 weeks of treatment in those who respond to sodium cromoglycate. If there is no response, a deterioration in the clinical state or the severity of the asthma was underestimated, sodium cromoglycate should be withdrawn and an inhaled corticosteroid introduced. For sodium cromoglycate to work, the bronchial inflammation should not be so severe that there is persistent mucosal oedema and a productive cough. In this situation, the use of sodium cromoglycate or an inhaled corticosteroid is inappropriate. Such severe inflammation should be suppressed with a short course of systemic steroids before preventive therapy is started. It is essential that preventive agents maintain maximum penetration, otherwise small areas of inflammation will persist and cause further hyperreactivity, even peripheral air trapping.

Inhaled corticosteroids are available in dry powder and aerosol preparations. Administration is twice daily, due to the long half lives of the drugs concerned (principally beclomethasone and budesonide). Before deciding upon the precise means of administration, i.e. a particular device, it is important to consider the points mentioned earlier, especially aiming to use the minimum effective dose. There is a wide variation in dosage between different children and between the ages of 4 and 16 years. Budesonide is available only in aerosol inhalers; beclomethasone is available in 2 dry powder forms and in aerosol inhalers. The dry powder device is likely to achieve control on about twice the dosage applicable to an aerosol used with a Volumatic device. This is an important consideration to bear in mind if we remember that most of the long term growth studies were done when the original beclomethasone dipropionate aerosol was the only available preparation, so that smaller doses up to 600 μg were inevitably used.

The most common dosage of beclomethasone dipropionate via an inhaler is 200 μg, twice daily, and with a dry powder device it is likely to be 400 μg, twice daily. Inhaled corticosteroid therapy demonstrates a flexible response; doses cannot be rigidly fixed but should be kept to a minimum so that an asymptomatic state or as near as possible, is maintained. It is important that adjustments to dosage, notably reductions, are made in a planned and informed fashion after a period of stability. This same flexibility will also allow the dosage to be temporarily increased in the presence of a particularly strong provoking factor, such as a heavy allergen load or a viral infection; in this situation the dosage can be safely doubled to contain the inflammatory response. As stated elsewhere, the adult shows a biochemical recognition of beclomethasone dipropionate therapy at a daily dosage of 1000 – 1600 μg and this dose might be crudely extrapolated to children and adolescents. It is tempting to resort to inhaled corticosteroids as a short cut to efficacy, but they are not always appropriate or necessary as a first line treatment. On some occasions, such a course will be appropriate, taking into account the factors mentioned elsewhere.

Nedocromil sodium has a product licence for use in children over 12 years of age. Its role will become clear in time, but it might be tried in those over 12 years of age who have problems with oropharyngeal thrush on inhaled corticosteroids. It is available only as an aerosol and can be used directly or via a Nebuhaler, taking 2 puffs (4 mg) 2 to 4 times daily. If it proves to have a safety profile comparable with that of sodium cromoglycate, it will perhaps be used as an intermediate therapy between sodium cromoglycate and inhaled corticosteroids in the young.

Controlled reduction or withdrawal of therapy should be considered if prophylaxis is successful and an asymptomatic period ocurs that covers an individual's trigger periods, such as infections in winter or airborne allergens in summer. If there have been symptom breakthroughs, it is best not to consider this approach. Even when therapy is withdrawn, it is commonly needed at a later date.

The asthma of only a very small minority of children cannot be controlled with the treatment detailed here. The most common cause of failure is the lack of compliance with therapy. This problem must be tackled in a sensitive fashion. The patient–doctor relationship has to survive honest inquiries. This relationship is more likely to be sustained if the GP has made it obvious that he or she has the patient's best interests at heart. For the tiny number of children who still have nocturnal symptoms after all our efforts, a slow-release theophylline preparation can be tried (*see* p. 87). Since the advent of inhaled corticosteroids, very few children now need maintenance systemic corticosteroids.

Acute severe asthma

If symptoms increase in severity despite therapy, but a bronchodilator restores the PEFR to the previous best level, inhaled preventive therapy may be doubled in dosage to overcome the increased bronchial hyperreactivity. If this fails, a course of prednisolone (1 – 2 mg/kg/day up to 20 mg and 0.6 mg/kg/day in adolescents) will be indicated until normality has been restored, after which long term therapy may need to be reviewed.

It is imperative that patients recognize when their asthma is deteriorating. They must be alert to progressively increasing symptoms that require repeated doses of bronchodilators which do not completely relieve their symptoms. Those patients who have a peak flow meter at home will be aware of a falling PEFR that never returns to its previous levels, even after inhalation of a bronchodilator. Deterioration must not be allowed to continue unchecked.

We should not be seeing patients who have had many successive nights disturbed by asthma, who are hardly able to walk because of breathlessness, and who may not be able to lie down either. The important signs are similar to those in younger children.

- Severe breathlessness.
- Raised respiratory rate (>30 breaths/minute).
- Raised heart rate ($>110 - 120$ beats/minute).
- Use of accessory muscles of respiration.
- Over-inflated chest.
- Increased wheeze, perhaps resulting in a 'silent' chest.
- PEFR $<50\%$ of usual level and not rising significantly after inhalation of bronchodilator.
- Such severe dyspnoea that there is insufficient time and breath to activate adequately a dry-powder device or co-ordinate with an aerosol inhaler, and thus the concentration of agent received falls drastically.

- Cyanosis.
- Difficulty in speaking.
- Difficulty in co-ordinating drinking and breathing, leading to dehydration.
- Exhaustion.

All these points should be taken into consideration in the overall assessment of severity. An often quoted but rarely measured phenomenon is the pulsus paradoxus which is most easily detected clinically by the disappearance of the peripheral pulse during inspiration. This sign is not always present, even in severe asthma, but the 'degree of paradox' can be measured by monitoring the blood pressure. As the mercury column falls the first sounds are heard only during expiration; as it falls further, the sounds are also heard during inspiration, the difference between the two being the degree of paradox. Values in excess of 15 mmHg are considered to be significant.

Clinical evaluation should confirm that the trachea is not deviated and that chest wall excursions are symmetrical. If dyspnoea is disproportionately severe, the patient is more ill than his symptoms of asthma alone would account for, and if there are signs of mediastinal shift and reduced breath sounds on one side, a pneumothorax should be suspected and arrangements made for an immediate chest X-ray.

Severe asthma must be treated promptly and vigorously. The heart rate, respiratory rate and PEFR must be assessed before administering treatment. A nebulized beta$_2$-agonist is required, with salbutamol in a Nebule in a dosage of 2.5 – 5 mg or as respirator solution diluted with normal saline, or terbutaline in a dosage of 5 mg as a Respule, or 5 – 10 mg in diluted respirator solution. Prednisolone may be administered orally, in a dosage of up to 40 mg, according to the child's age and weight. If the child is very ill or is vomiting, hydrocortisone in a dosage of 100 – 200 μg is given intravenously.

The child's general clinical condition and PEFR are reviewed after the nebulized bronchodilator therapy. It is important not to rely upon the subjective, partly placebo response to nebulized therapy. As with the younger child the nebulized treatment is repeated initially every 2 hours. Those who are very ill, who require close observation, oxygen therapy with blood gas monitoring and in whom even assisted ventilation may be necessary, require hospitalization.

Occasionally, perhaps in the absence of a nebulizer, the first dose of beta$_2$-agonist can be given intravenously (for dosage, *see* p. 79). Intravenous aminophylline has no place today as a first line emergency therapy. Those patients in whom it might be used are more likely to be on long acting oral preparations of theophylline which makes intravenous administration very dangerous.

Ensure that nebulizer – respirator solutions are not used for intravenous administration.

Those patients not responding to the therapy within 6 – 8 hours should be reassessed for admission to hospital. For those who do respond, the intervals between nebulizer use can be progressively lengthened up to once every 6 hours before switching to a lower dose form of therapy, such as dry powder or by Nebuhaler.

The dosage of prednisolone is maintained until lung function returns to normal, as judged by symptoms, signs and measurements such as PEFR. At this point, the introduction of preventive therapy should be considered; this is an easy decision if it is part of a recurring pattern. If there has been a build up to this acute or subacute deterioration, systemic steroids will need to be tailed off after 1 – 2 weeks, with the introduction of preventive therapy to maintain effective suppression of the inflammation. In this situation it is important to review the treatment and the patient's need for it constantly. It is sensible after one severe episode to suppress bronchial inflammation for about 3 months with a prophylactic agent, then to review the situation with the patient. The patient must regard the GP's advice as justifiable and appropriate.

In summary

Acute severe asthma

Inhaled bronchodilator:

Terbutaline— < 25 kg body-weight (about 8 years) 5 – 10 puffs (1.25 – 2.5 mg) via Nebuhaler over 15 minutes every 2 – 6 hours, or 3 – 5 mg (0.3 – 0.5 ml) as respirator solution diluted to 2 ml with normal saline, via nebulizer; > 25 kg 10 – 20 puffs (2.5 – 5 mg) via Nebuhaler or 5 mg in 2 ml as Respule.

Salbutamol— 2.5 – 5 mg in Nebules (2.5 ml) or by dilution of respirator solution with normal saline, via nebulizer.

Systemic corticosteroid:

Prednisolone—1 – 2 mg/kg/day up to 20 mg/day, then 0.6 mg/kg for older children (but rather empirical) up to 30 – 40 mg, as tablets or soluble tablets.

Hydrocortisone sodium succinate—100 – 200 mg i.v. if the patient is very ill or vomiting.

Preventive therapy:

Sodium cromoglycate—1 – 2 puffs (5 – 10 mg) 4 or more times daily perhaps via a Nebuhaler or Spincaps 20 mg, 4 or more times daily in a Spinhaler.

Nedocromil sodium—>12 years, 2 puffs (4 mg) twice or four times daily, from a metered dose inhaler or via Nebuhaler.

Beclomethasone—perhaps 100 – 200 μg, twice daily either directly from a metered dose inhaler or via Volumatic or 200 – 400 μg, twice daily by dry powder device.

Budesonide— 50 – 200 μg, twice daily, either directly from a metered dose inhaler or via Nebuhaler.

Treatment of asthma in adult life

Adult asthma sufferers are generally either:

1 atopic individuals whose asthma has come and gone or persisted since childhood, or which has appeared later, perhaps in association with hay fever or other seasonal allergies; or
2 those individuals who have developed late onset asthma from middle age onwards, with no allergic associations.

Those atopic asthmatics with intermittent symptoms will need occasional treatment, whereas those with persistent asthma from childhood and those who have late onset asthma will need long term preventive therapy.

Although a patient's rate of growth is no longer a consideration, it is essential that adult asthma sufferers do not gain weight with age, because obesity causes diaphragmatic restriction, especially when the patient bends over. Weight gain and obesity may be a problem for some late onset asthmatics who may need to take occasional or regular courses of systemic corticosteroids, which will add to the weight problem. A weight reducing diet may be highly beneficial in this situation.

Other changes related to age should be borne in mind when prescribing:

1 a change in the metabolism of theophyllines;
2 an exaggeration of benign essential tremor, especially by oral preparations but even by inhaled beta$_2$-agonists;
3 the regular use of corticosteroids may precipitate hypertension or diabetes mellitus in those subjects who are susceptible.

Basic relief of symptoms and preventive therapy

The atopic asthmatic is less likely to suffer from exercise-induced symptoms in adult life, because he or she is less likely to indulge in vigorous exercise. However, before exercise-induced symptoms become a regular feature, the asthma will tend to have increased in severity and chronicity. Once exercise-induced asthma has become established, the threshold for provocation is very low. The treatment for occasional provoked symptoms in an essentially stable situation is an inhaled beta$_2$-agonist, either via a dry powder device or a metered dose inhaler.

Seasonal asthma is fairly common in the adult atopic asthmatic. Its occurrence can usually be predicted. Symptoms appear at a similar time each year, between spring and autumn, which may vary slightly according to weather conditions. The severity will also vary: sometimes only mild daytime exercise-induced asthma occurs, but, more commonly, there is unprovoked asthma in the evening and early hours of the morning. Although a beta$_2$-agonist might appear to be adequate treatment in some cases, it should be remembered that in about 50% the asthma will be a manifestation of the late asthmatic response. Thus it is clear that the use of a prophylactic agent is necessary, backed up by a beta$_2$-agonist, if required. As in adolescence, the choice is between sodium cromoglycate, nedocromil sodium or inhaled corticosteroids in the usual dosages. Therapy should be started at the first sign of asthma or in anticipation of the season's events.

More persistent asthma, whether atopic or of late onset, should be treated with a combination of bronchodilators and prophylactic agents. Some patients show a marked response to bronchodilator therapy, which occasionally appears to be of relatively short duration (2 – 3 hours) in the absence of a significant steroid response. Anticholinergic bronchodilators, such as ipratropium, have an increased role in adult asthmatics, in conjunction with beta$_2$-agonists. However, the response to bronchodilators cannot always be predicted and, so that therapy can be tailored to each individual patient, a trial of response should be made, either clinically or as a reversibility test.

A typical dose of salbutamol is 1 or 2 puffs (100 – 200 μg) 2 – 4 times daily, depending upon need, via an aerosol inhaler. With increased age some patients suffer from poor co-ordination—they may cope with a Rotahaler or Diskhaler, although clumsy or trembling fingers find it difficult to load them. In some patients, unless salbutamol were to be taken via a Volumatic, the Turbohaler might be more acceptable because it is easier to operate, simply requiring a twisting action to prime it. The Turbohaler dispenses terbutaline 500 μg, compared with 250 μg in the aerosol presentation. With salbutamol, some patients will require doses as high as 1600 μg (4 $\times$ 400 μg Rotacaps), 4 or more times daily.

Ipratropium is available for administration only via the aerosol inhaler in two dosages—18 and 36 μg per puff; the usual dosage is 1 – 2 puffs (36 – 72 μg) 3 or 4 times daily. It will usually complement the action of the beta$_2$-agonist.

For those atopic asthmatics with seasonal symptoms, sodium cromoglycate is likely to remain as the prophylactic agent of first choice. However, late onset asthmatics and those atopic asthmatics who have suffered chronic asthma from childhood and adolescence are likely to require therapy with nedocromil sodium or inhaled corticosteroids. As stated earlier, nedocromil sodium may be equivalent in effect to low dose inhaled steroids in the range of up to perhaps 400 μg of beclomethasone per day. Late onset asthma is often more difficult to control, requiring higher dose therapy and sometimes maintenance systemic corticosteroids due to the condition itself or to a past history of tobacco smoking or an adverse working environment.

The dosage of inhaled steroids will vary considerably; for example, beclomethasone dosages range from 200 μg twice daily via aerosol inhaler, to 750 – 1000 μg twice daily from a high dose inhaler. Such doses will be more effectively administered by a large volume spacer, such as a Volumatic in the case of beclomethasone. Those who use dry powder devices, such as the Rotahaler or Diskhaler, will take beclomethasone 400 – 1000 μg twice daily.

Despite good compliance with therapy, some older patients will require additional treatment, usually for nocturnal symptoms, but also to improve daytime control. The most commonly used supplementary drug is theophylline (for dosages, *see* page 87). There are several long acting theophylline preparations with different release characteristics which are not interchangeable dose for dose.

Transferring to a different preparation will necessitate restabilization, either by increasing or reducing the dosage, judged on clinical critera, with or without the estimation of serum levels. Theophyllines can be purchased without prescription and patients acquiring such medication may not inform their GP that they are taking it. This is a dangerous situation because if an additional theophylline is prescribed toxicity might occur.

Some patients may benefit from the use of sustained release beta$_2$-agonists such as Volmax (4 or 8 mg salbutamol), taken at night or twice daily.

A small proportion of patients may still need to take a small maintenance dose of prednisolone to maintain the suppression of the asthmatic process but there is always a difficult balance between the failure to treat and the side effects of long term treatment.

Acute severe asthma

Mortality from asthma is higher in adults. Many adults will tolerate the most appalling symptoms without consulting a GP. Some severe asthmatics remain undiagnosed, either because they do not present or because the GP fails to recognize asthma because of the clinical picture associated with age. Correctly diagnosed asthmatics who are receiving treatment may fail to notice the warning signs of deteriorating asthma or they may be inappropriately treated with antibiotics when they require high dose systemic corticosteroids.

The warning signs are similar to those that occur in childhood and adolescence (*see* p. 126), but the patient's ability to cope may be less, due to age. Adult asthmatics are often in a worse clinical state than younger asthmatics. The effects of smoking on the lungs and the heart will also have been detrimental.

Those asthmatics already receiving treatment should be aware of the indications of deterioration, such as nocturnal disturbances, increased and less effective bronchodilator consumption and a falling PEFR. At an early stage of symptomatic deterioration (a fall in PEFR of about 25% which is largely reversible), it may be possible to double inhaled preventive and bronchodilator therapy temporarily. If this manoeuvre fails or the PEFR falls to individually set levels, prompt, energetic measures need to be taken. A patient with a good understanding of events can initiate corticosteroid therapy and increase the bronchodilator dosage before calling the GP. If obstruction increases significantly and reduces the inspiratory capacity, a large volume spacer and an aerosol inhaler are useful. When the dosage of inhaled steroid is increased to prevent an exacerbation, it is often valuable to increase the frequency of administration to 3 or 4 times daily.

Clinical assessment must take the overall clinical picture into account. Difficulty in speaking, heart rate, respiratory rate and PEFR should be monitored before and after the administration of a nebulized beta$_2$-agonist, such as 5 – 10 mg of salbutamol (1 – 2 ml respirator solution diluted to 2.5 ml with normal saline). This should be accompanied by the administration of prednisolone, 0.6 mg/kg/day, typical doses being 30 – 60 mg. In the event of the patient being very ill or vomiting, hydrocortisone can be administered intravenously, in a dosage of 200 mg. I would have profound reservations about using intravenous aminophylline for the reasons mentioned earlier. If available, oxygen could be given between nebulized therapies, but any patient who requires oxygen should be admitted to hospital. In the presence of marked obstruction with mucus plugging the intravenous route for beta$_2$-agonist therapy with salbutamol or terbutaline is indicated. Some patients show a greater response if nebulized ipratropium is used with the beta$_2$-agonist (250 – 500 μg in 1 – 2 ml).

If the patient is well enough to be treated at home and home circumstances permit, it is necessary to review the patient within 2 hours and probably repeat the nebulized beta$_2$-agonist, with or without ipratropium. Although it is unlikely that a very 'obstructed' asthmatic will absorb sufficient beta$_2$-agonist to precipitate a tachydysrhythmia, it is possible that one might occur as the patient's condition improves, before the dosage of beta$_2$-agonist and the interval between treatments have been reduced. In the older patient, the GP must be alert to the onset of tachycardia and consequent myocardial ischaemia.

The presence of dyspepsia should indicate the possibility of steroid induced peptic ulceration which itself warrants treatment with an H_2-antagonist for example. There is significant morbidity, and sometimes mortality, associated with peptic ulceration in patients who have severe asthma.

Antibiotics should be used only if there is a suggestion of bacterial infection, such as pyrexia, localizing chest signs and 'purulent' sputum.

The dosage of prednisolone is maintained until airflow obstruction has been reversed and a stable state attained. This may take 2 weeks or more if there has been a long history of asthma. If the patient has been kept at home or has been discharged from hospital early, it is advisable to carry out home monitoring of PEFR as either marked airways instability or secondary mucus obstruction may occur, both of which can delay recovery or have more serious consequences.

Based upon a consideration of previous history, previous treatment and the treatment response during this current episode, the corticosteroids can be stopped or reduced over days or weeks. Bronchodilator dosage can be reduced and the interval between doses extended to 6 hours.

Any patient who suffers a severe exacerbation of asthmatic symptoms should be educated further about asthma; how the treatment works and how to respond to certain danger signs. Although there will always be some patients who do not respond to this regimen, most patients will appreciate and act on such advice, particularly if it is reinforced on later visits. The patient needs to be aware that treatment is not random but planned to be as convenient as possible, while enabling them to gain the maximum therapeutic benefit possible.

In summary

Acute, severe asthma

Bronchodilator

Salbutamol— by nebulizer, 5 – 10 mg, either one Nebule or respirator solution, 1 – 2 ml, diluted with normal saline, every 2 – 6 hours.

Terbutaline— 5 – 10 mg, as 1 – 2 Respules or diluted respirator solution (0.5 – 1 ml).

Ipratropium—250 – 500 μg (1 – 2 ml) as nebulizer solution, diluted with normal saline, if necessary.

Corticosteroid

Prednisolone—0.6 mg/kg/day – 30 – 60 mg as plain, soluble or enteric-coated tablets (5 mg).

Hydrocortisone sodium succinate—200 mg intravenously, if the patient is very ill or vomiting.

Preventive therapy

Beclomethasone—200 – 1000 μg twice daily, by aerosol inhaler (± volumatic) or dry powder device.

Budesonide— 200 – 600 μg, twice daily, ± Nebuhaler.

Nedocromil sodium—4 mg (2 puffs) 2 to 4 times daily with or without a Nebuhaler.

Hay fever and perennial rhinitis

Hay fever is a common feature of atopy and often accompanies asthma. Perennial rhinitis suggests a related problem, predominantly affecting the nose, which persists throughout the year.

Management can be approached in two ways:

1 Antihistamines can be taken, usually by mouth, although topical preparations are available. Personally, I prefer not to prescribe topical antihistamines (eye drops, etc.) because of the risk of sensitization. Antihistamines compete at the histamine receptors with histamine itself, to block the mediator's effects. Currently, there is an increasing number of H_1-antagonists that do not have such marked sedative effects. Some can be taken once daily, such as astemizole 10 mg, cetirizine 10 mg, terphenadine 120 mg and loratadine 10 mg, and others are taken 3 times daily, such as acrivastine 8 mg. They all counter allergic rhinitis, conjunctivitis and urticaria but do not completely alleviate the symptoms for all hay fever sufferers.

2 Local agents can be used to reduce the allergic inflammatory reaction in the nasal and conjunctival mucosae. In my experience, sodium cromoglycate eye drops, in an aqueous form (4 times daily), are the safest, most effective therapy for allergic conjunctivitis. They probably act by reducing mast cell degranulation and reducing the cellular infiltrate.

The most effective agents for nasal problems, whether seasonal or perennial, are nasal topical steroid preparations, either aqueous or aerosol, although the latter may cause mucosal drying. Examples are budesonide, beclomethasone and flunisolide. These preparations should be applied twice daily to each nostril as preventive agents. Nasal preparations of sodium cromoglycate are also available. In patients with perennial rhinitis and asthma, the effective treatment of a blocked and discharging/secreting nose will often help the asthma, especially at night. On exceptional occasions, when all other treatment has been ineffective, steroid injections, lasting 3 – 6 weeks, may be administered, for example Depo-Medrone (methylprednisolone) 40 – 80 mg in 1 – 2 ml i.m.

Eczema

The appearance of eczema is not reliably associated with asthma, but the two conditions often coexist. The severe pruritus often associated with eczema is most effectively relieved by mild to moderate strength topical corticosteroids. Emollients and tar based remedies are largely ineffective in active inflammation.

Therapy used wisely is safe, but potent topical steroids should be avoided on the face and used only on the rest of the body for as long as is necessary before they are tailed off. Emollients should be applied in the interim.

Occasionally there are obvious dietary associations, but this is not usually the case, and children in particular should not be placed on inadequate diets in the hope of finding the factor responsible for the eczema.

Illustrative case histories

Adam

Adam was brought to the surgery when he was 2½ years old. He had developed a cough at night, which initially disturbed only his parents. Now he was being woken by it, somewhat distressed, breathless and with a hint of a wheeze. He had also started to cough a good deal when he ran about at his toddler group. There was a strong family history of asthma and Adam had had infantile eczema from the age of 6 months. There were no abnormal findings when he was examined in the surgery and Adam was perfectly well between attacks, thus tending to confirm mother's strong suspicion that he had asthma.

The diagnosis and treatment were discussed with Adam's mother—the nocturnal cough was a manifestation of bronchial hyperreactivity—and the proposed course of action was to try to suppress the mild inflammatory reaction in the bronchi with sodium cromoglycate. Means of administration can be a problem at Adam's age but he was able to master a Nebuhaler, through which he took sodium cromoglycate, 5 mg (1 puff) 4 times daily. He was also prescribed a terbutaline inhaler to use if the asthma symptoms broke through. On this regimen, his asthma was well controlled until the age of 4½ years, when he started school and had a succession of 'colds' that precipitated quite severe asthma. He was now taking sodium cromoglycate by Spinhaler, 20 mg 4 times daily. Although the dosage was increased at the first hint of a cold, it failed to control the asthma and he finally needed a course of Prednesol and nebulized salbutamol, as 2.5 mg Nebules.

A review of Adam's treatment led to the prescription of beclomethasone Rotacaps, 200 μg, 1, twice daily after a salbutamol Rotacap, 200 μg, which he could also use if he experienced occasional exercise-induced symptoms. Adam's mother again reported good control of his asthma; if the dose of this preventive therapy was doubled at the beginning of a cold, his asthma remained suppressed. The inhaled steroid could have been given by a large volume spacer, but in the interests of consistency both agents were taken as a dry powder.

Giles and James

The case histories of Giles and James illustrate the differences in care that have taken place between the birth of James in 1979 and that of Giles in 1985.

James had begun to get wheezy with 'colds' by the time he was 16 months old. By the age of 2 years he had been unwell on several occasions and was being treated with intermittent nebulized salbutamol 2.5 mg in 2.5 ml (made up from respirator solution) and antibiotics on occasions when he was febrile. By 2 years and 3 months, he had received his first course of prednisolone (15 mg/day). He was admitted to hospital on several occasions over the next 3 years, and was provided with a home nebulizer by the hospital staff. He was 5 years old (October 1984) before anyone prescribed an inhaled prophylactic agent for him—beclomethasone as Rotacaps. The greatest hurdle thenceforth was to convince James's mother it was better to treat him with a regular preventive agent that would keep James well, rather than resort to intervention in a succession of crises superimposed on his chronic symptoms.

Despite the fact that James's mother smokes heavily at home, which James detests, his asthma is now very well controlled on inhaled salbutamol and beclomethasone, as Rotacaps, 400 μg of each drug twice daily. He has had no prednisolone for 18 months. His height and PEFR are average for his age.

Giles developed his first wheeze with a cold when he was 3 months old. As there were older children in the family, it seemed inevitable that a new respiratory virus entered the home every 2 weeks. Giles's symptoms became almost chronic and he was failing to thrive—the possibility of cystic fibrosis was excluded. He was admitted to hospital at the age of 13 months where it was found that he had a response to nebulized ipratropium. Nebulized salbutamol had no effect before Giles was 18 months old, but he was kept almost free of symptoms for 3 months with nebulized sodium cromoglycate and occasional ipratropium. Over the next 6 months, he had 2 severe exacerbations and was again admitted to hospital. At almost 2 years of age, it was decided to try and treat him with beclomethasone (50 μg) 2 puffs, 3 times daily through a Volumatic device, after 2 puffs of salbutamol on each occasion; on this regimen, he has had no exacerbations of his asthma for over 12 months.

These case histories demonstrate that both the drugs and their delivery systems must be tailored to each patient.

Mick

Mick is a 26 year old non-smoking lorry driver who is married with two young children. He has had asthma since childhood and until recently it was controlled by sodium cromoglycate Spincaps, 20 mg 4 times daily, and occasional salbutamol. Mick is now being woken every night by his symptoms; much of the day his PEFR is about 400 l/min with little provocation and he has only a partial response to bronchodilator therapy.

Due to this persistent obstruction, Mick was treated with systemic corticosteroids, 40 mg of prednisolone daily, until his asthma was stable and he could be put onto a beclomethasone inhaler, 200 μg twice daily after his salbutamol. Although his asthma remained well controlled, he developed intractable, unacceptable oral thrush despite amphotericin lozenges and use of a large volume spacer, the Volumatic. He was changed to an inhaler containing nedocromil sodium, starting on 2 puffs twice daily and increasing to 4 puffs twice daily (which was more convenient than 2 puffs 4 times daily). This regimen has controlled Mick's asthma and has not given rise to oral thrush.

Malcolm

Malcolm is 27 years old, overweight and suffers from Down's syndrome. He is not atopic and has had no serious illnesses but he was very breathless and cyanosed when he was seen during the course of an acute illness which was associated with a cough and shortness of breath. Admitted to hospital, he was correctly diagnosed as having atypical pneumonia, with bilateral consolidation. He made a slow recovery on antibiotic therapy. A follow up chest X-ray was normal. Six months later he developed a cough and became cyanosed; he was re-admitted to hospital. The cyanosis was thought to be secondary to a right-to-left shunt precipitated by the respiratory infection. On this occasion, overall recovery was incomplete in that Malcolm experienced disturbing nocturnal symptoms that were difficult to describe but could have been either sleep apnoea or airway obstruction associated with his obesity. The pattern then developed in which he woke regularly, breathless and wheezing.

Once shown, he was able to use a peak flow meter very easily, which demonstrated the following:

1 his daytime PEFR rose from 420 to 500 l/min after inhalation of salbutamol from a Volumatic;
2 his PEFR at night fell to 300 l/min.

A diagnosis of asthma was made, perhaps precipitated by the infections. He was started on a treatment regimen of a salbutamol inhaler, 2 puffs, twice daily, followed by beclomethasone 100 μg, 2 puffs twice daily via a Volumatic, with extra salbutamol as required. The effect has been remarkable; his inhalation technique is impeccable, he has had no symptoms for 18 months and his PEFR is 700 l/min.

Albert

Albert is retired and 68 years old. At the age of 51 years he had nasal polyps removed and from then on he suffered from repeated episodes of 'bronchitis', usually in the winter but occasionally in the summer (2 – 3 times each year). He gave up pipe smoking 6 years ago. Four years ago his PEFR was 350 l/min when recovering from further bronchitis after 'flu'.

This spring Albert presented with a bad cough and a wheeze at night and a feeling of tightness across his chest. An ECG was normal. His chest was wheezy with rattles at the lung bases; his PEFR was 380 l/min and his chest X-ray showed mild non-specific inflammatory appearances at the bases. From his current and past histories and the clinical findings, a diagnosis of asthma was made.

He was started on prednisolone 30 mg daily and salbutamol Rotacaps 2 × 400 μg, 4 times daily. Within 18 days, he had improved to his 'best for ages', with no phlegm and a PEFR of up to 475 l/min. He has now been taken off prednisolone; the dosage was reduced slowly over 4 weeks. He is maintained on salbutamol Rotacaps 400 μg, 1 twice daily followed by beclomethasone 400 μg Rotacaps, twice daily, with extra salbutamol if needed. In retrospect, Albert says he feels a different person.

The organization of care

The modern management of asthma and other chronic disorders demands a new approach. Due to the nature of conditions such as asthma, diabetes mellitus and hypertension and the therapeutic agents previously available, their management was determined by symptomatic demand and concentrated upon crisis intervention in hospitals and general practice.

The past 20 years have witnessed great changes: diabetic patients can now monitor their condition at home and adjust insulin dosage; hypertensive subjects can have their blood pressure returned to physiological levels, thus averting long term damage to the cardiovascular system. The advent of these novel management techniques has dramatically reduced the once regular admissions for recurrent hypoglycaemia and ketoacidosis, and the attendant morbidity and mortality, and the need to reduce the blood pressure in malignant hypertension by titrating the blood pressure against doses of potent hypotensive agents, occasionally with catastrophic results.

Most medical students, student nurses, young doctors and nurses regard asthma as an acute condition which they will have treated with intravenous bronchodilators, nebulized bronchodilators and large doses of systemic corticosteroids. They may have little knowledge of the daily symptoms and regular nocturnal disturbances which may go unreported. Often, they will not witness or take part in the planning of long term preventive therapy of patients with asthma. They may have an awareness of prophylactic agents but little experience of their use.

This scheme of crisis intervention is reinforced by the misuse of the admirable concept of self referral devised for severe asthmatics who are prone to suffer severe life threatening exacerbations of asthma despite regular prophylactic therapy. Self referral is planned so that the patient, thoracic unit, GP and the local ambulance headquarters are aware of the patients involved, to minimize delays in providing immediate care. Unfortunately, the concept has been misapplied, especially in the management of children with asthma. Children on inadequate or no prophylactic therapy are seen repeatedly on children's wards or in accident and emergency departments. Usually nebulized bronchodilator therapy is given and the patient is discharged home. Communication with the patient's GP is inadequate and there is no cohesive plan for the management of that patient's asthma. Repeated acute attacks indicate unstable asthma, which is dangerous.

The place for asthma care is in general practice. One has only to consider the numbers to appreciate that in my Health Authority, each general practitioner has 100 – 125 current asthmatics on his list, while our single chest physician is responsible for 12,500! Hardly a viable proposition to treat the bulk of asthma in our hospitals.

The regular use of prophylactic therapy in asthma will reduce the occurrence of exacerbations and allow a normal lifestyle for the majority of subjects with uncomplicated asthma. However, long term therapy demands that the patient is followed up for several reasons.

1 As the patient is using pharmacologically active agents, his or her general well being should be monitored.
2 The effectiveness of the therapy should be assessed.
3 The patient's understanding of asthma and its treatment should be revised and inhaler techniques examined.
4 The patient's need for therapy should be reassessed.
5 The patient's knowledge of what to do in the event of an acute exacerbation should be reviewed and reinforced.
6 The need for, or the results of, PEFR home monitoring should be considered.

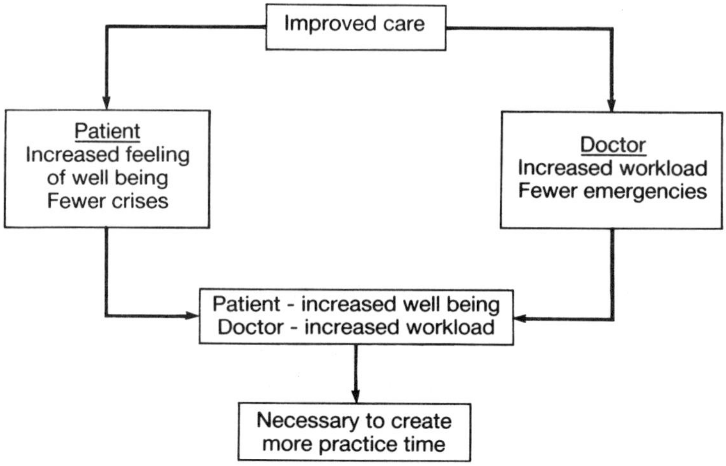

Figure 8.7 Asthma care equation.

This may seem rather tame when compared with treating emergencies but we need to learn to gain quiet professional satisfaction from the restoration of a normal life, without awaiting the next case of acute severe asthma.

It would be naïve to believe that the time saved from responding to asthmatic emergencies would compensate for the time required for the planned, anticipatory care of asthma (Fig. 8.7). Whether in hospital or in general practice, the preventive care of a symptomatic disorder will take a considerable amount of time, especially in the early days. The requirements of anticipatory care are:

1 adequate diagnosis;
2 full assessment of the asthma;
3 rational treatment tailored to the individual and the situation;
4 planned follow up and reassessment;
5 intervention, with adjustment of therapy, when appropriate;
6 patient and family education;
7 good rapport with the patient and his or her family.

It is essential that follow up should not simply be a case of recording symptoms and home PEFR measurements, supplemented by an examination and PEFR or spirometry at the time of the consultation. The follow up is a time for reassessment.

- Is there a repeated breakthrough of symptoms?
- If so, is the PEFR also unstable with marked oscillations?

- In the presence of recurrent symptoms and the absence of PEFR home monitoring, should a peak flow meter be provided?
- Is the therapy adequate or appropriate?
- Is therapy being taken regularly, or is the return of symptoms related to poor compliance?
- If there is poor compliance, what is the cause?
- Does the patient understand when and why to take the medication?
- If compliance is good, does the treatment need to be altered or supplemented?

The aim of asthma care for the majority of patients is to provide a base from which they can become relatively self sufficient, with expert advice and support from their GPs. An important component of this is patient education. However, it is dangerous to assume that, once provided with background information on asthma and its treatment, all patients will be self reliant thereafter. Patient education requires constant reinforcement. Unless repeated regularly, patients forget facts and techniques. If 40 and 15 minutes are allowed for both assessment and follow up, I have estimated that to review all current asthmatics in an average practice and to carry out one follow up visit would add 8% to the practice workload in the first year of such a programme. After the first year, the time commitment is for newly diagnosed asthmatics and follow up of those who are already known, which will be a little less than 8%.

It is important to structure the follow up, otherwise subsequent consultations may become ineffective head nodding encounters from which the patient derives no benefit. The GP must allow adequate time for an initial, thorough assessment and for follow up visits.

When the principles of diagnosis and treatment are well understood, any new treatments should be made available if appropriate.

We must accept the need to create extra practice time and the GP(s) concerned will need to consider whether to care for asthmatics themselves or to recruit help from within the practice team. Any programme for improved care will need to be GP based, and to use the GP's expertise in asthma care, *see* Fig. 8.7.

Teamwork in asthma care

In our practice we have shown that an appropriately trained nurse can undertake much of the routine care of asthmatic patients, in conjunction with the GP(s). Such a programme will evolve slowly as the nurse gains in practical experience and for individual patients the proportion of the work and responsibility carried out by the doctor and nurse will vary tremendously. The nurse's involvement may be illustrated as follows.

A graded role for the nurse in asthma care

Zero involvement—Patient sees only the GP.

Minimum involvement—Patient always sees the GP.

Nurse may:

1 set up an asthma register;
2 measure and record PEFR;
3 demonstrate, instruct and check on inhalation techniques.

Medium involvement—Potential for a joint GP/nurse clinic.

Nurse may:

4 carry out further tests (for example, reversibility, exercise);
5 teach PEFR home monitoring and the use of diary cards;
6 improve asthma education;
7 provide explanatory literature.

Maximum involvement—Nurse-run clinic with GP availability and review.

Nurse may:

8 carry out full assessments and regular follow up;
9 formulate a structured treatment plan, in conjunction with the GP and the patient;
10 write prescriptions to be signed by the GP;
11 give telephone advice where appropriate;
12 see patients in an 'emergency', that is presentation with increased or renewed symptoms.

A Separate Clinic?

A fundamental decision when organizing the care of asthmatics is whether separate time is devoted to asthma or whether to fit it into normal consulting sessions. This depends very much on practice organization. It is not always possible to know when a given patient has asthma, especially if they are presenting for the first time. If tests to confirm diagnosis, such as exercise and reversibility tests, are performed during the time (10 min) normally allotted to the consultation, the disruption can be considerable. To have these tests supervised by the nurse can be invaluable.

Since adopting this separate clinic approach it has become apparent that it is not important who manages asthma, provided it is managed well. This requires the doctor and the nurse to be well informed about asthma. In order to plan care it is necessary to fulfil the following requirements.

1 A nurse should be specially trained and well motivated.
2 A doctor with a special interest in asthma should oversee the running of the clinic.
3 A register of the practice's asthma patients should be kept. It helps with strategic planning and audit, as well as allowing overall surveillance.
4 A structured plan for diagnosis and treatment should be laid out. It needs to be used as a guideline by all members of the team. An inconsistent approach causes confusion for the patient and for other members of the team. Inconsistency is a common cause of diminished confidence in members of the practice team.
5 It is important to allot time for patient education.
6 An effective recording system should be instituted. In order to obtain a consistent outcome and to make a patient's current status and therapy easily available. We have adopted an asthma card (which fits inside the FP5/FP6 folder) which has been designed to provide a more thorough history as well as recording current information (Fig. 8.8).
7 There should be arrangements for direct follow up. One great weakness of follow up is the strong likelihood of patients slipping through the net. This is less likely to occur if the patient makes an appointment *before* leaving the doctor or nurse.
8 Adequate space must be designated for the clinic. Although the GP is likely to have a consulting room already, the nurse will also need one. It is unsatisfactory to attempt to run a clinic in a busy treatment room if dressings and other procedures are being carried out at the same time. In addition, there is a need for telephone access to speak to patients or relatives and to advise on management when this is appropriate.

Running a Clinic

The following scheme might provide a framework for an asthma clinic within a general practice; it has been designed to produce a structured management plan for each individual patient, whoever provides the care. Points that refer specifically to nurse run asthma clinics (NRAC) are in italic type.

1 Compile a register of all known asthmatic subjects within the practice. This can be done from repeat prescriptions, GPs' lists, memory triggers

ASTHMA CLINIC - RECORD CARD

Name .... Sex ....

Address .... Marital status ....

.... Dr's name ....

Date of birth ....

INITIAL ASSESSMENT

Date ....

ASTHMATIC HISTORY

Year of onset of symptoms ☐☐☐☐

Year of asthma diagnosis ☐☐☐☐

Age at asthma diagnosis ☐☐

Family history ....

Occupational history ....

Eczema *(please put Y or N as appropriate in all following boxes)* ☐

Hay fever ☐

Urticaria ☐

Wheezy bronchitis ☐

Drug allergies ☐

Specify ....

PROVOCATION

Exercise ☐

Cold air ☐

Respiratory infection ☐

Emotion ☐

Cough/sneeze ☐

Laugh ☐

Work related ☐

Animals ☐

Seasonal element ☐

Specify season ....

....

....

PRESENT SYMPTOMS

Respiratory infection ☐

Sputum ☐

Cough ☐

If Y, specify Night or Day ....

Wheezy ☐

If Y specify worse time ....

....

ASTHMA STATE

Persistent ☐

Episodic ☐

CONTINUE ON BACK OF CARD

ASTHMA TREATMENT *(include oral & inhaled steroid therapy)*

Previous ....

....

....

Current ....

....

....

Other medical conditions & drug therapy

....

....

....

INVESTIGATIONS

Height: cms ☐☐☐ ft. ins. ☐☐ ☐☐

Weight: Kg. ☐☐☐ st. lbs. ☐☐ ☐☐

Smoking (Y or N) ☐

If Y, how many? ☐

If ever, when stopped ☐☐ ☐

and how many? ☐

Blood pressure (adults only) ....

Urine (if patient taking oral steroids: Glu .... .Prot ....

If requested: Hb ☐☐ · ☐ Skin tests ....

CXR ....

EDUCATION

Present level of understanding: High/Med/Low

Booklet given (Y or N) ☐

COMMENTS AND PLANS

....

....

....

FOR LUNG FUNCTION TESTS SEE INSIDE

Date	Time	Specify assessment, pre/post B'dilation, exercise test, etc.	Wright PEF Meas.	Wright PEF Pred.	Inhalation Technique	Comp	SYMPTOMS: (Always check symptoms against the following list: cough, respiratory infection, bronchitis, sputum, exercise-induced asthma. Wheeziness worse at night and first thing in morning?) **HOME CHARTING RESULTS, EDUCATION, PLANS & THERAPY.**	APPT.

(Comp ≡ compliance)

Figure 8.8 Asthma clinic record card.

or case finding. The patients thus identified will tend to be current asthmatics; those who have suffered from asthma previously can be added to the register as they are picked out later. It is useful to separate current from previous sufferers. One person must co-ordinate the register. The patient's name, date of birth, sex, address and GP's name should be recorded on an index card, or 'asthma' added to the list of diagnoses on the patient's computer record.

2 Mark the records distinctively.
3 *For a NRAC, it is necessary to choose a means of selection and referral to the clinic.*
4 *Compile a separate register for NRAC patients.*

Initial assessment

Allow 30 – 40 minutes to gain the maximum benefit from an in depth, unhurried consultation. The GP/nurse and patient/parent will be assessing one another and building up a rapport.

5 Explain the purpose and structure of the consultation, which is designed to gain the maximum information in a reasonable amount of time.
6 Measure the patient's height and weight and record them. This is important for 2 reasons: to be able to calculate the mean predicted values for PEFR and spirometry; and to monitor a child's growth, an important indication of well being.
7 Measure PEFR and spirometry (if available) and record the results, which can then be compared with predicted values.
8 If the patient has symptoms or the PEFR is below predicted levels, carry out a bronchodilator reversibility test (*see* p. 72), after checking or instructing in inhaler technique (aerosol), with or without an expansion chamber, or a dry powder device).
9 During the 15 minute wait before PEFR can be measured again, complete the structured interview and examination.
   - Ascertain the patient's asthmatic history.
   - Determine the trigger factors—provocation.
   - Record the present symptoms.
   - Assess the 'asthma state' (for example, persistent or episodic).
   - Inquire about previous and current treatment for asthma.
   - Ask about other medical conditions and their therapy (e.g. beta-blockers).
   - Check recent investigations, e.g. chest X-ray, blood count (anaemia), blood pressure.

10 Measure PEFR again and perhaps refer to the diagnosis and treatment flow chart (Fig. 8.3, *see* 108 – 9).

11 Smoking history: patient or immediate family who may be in the same household—smoking by any member of the family should be strongly discouraged.
12 From the information gathered, begin to formulate a treatment strategy.
13 *Discuss the projected treatment plan with the patient's GP and possibly invite the GP to join the consultation.*
14 After ascertaining exactly what the patient's concept of asthma is, explain about asthma in simple terms. Introduce and discuss the proposed treatment. However, do not overwhelm the patient or the family with too much detailed information during this first consultation. Try to give direct answers to searching questions.
15 Provide the patient or parent with:

- the relevant treatment card (Fig. 8.9, pages 147 – 9) which is partly pre-printed and then completed with written dosage instructions;
- booklet(s) on asthma;
- illustrated inhaler instructions;
- a mini peak flow meter and chart, if home monitoring of PEFR is necessary;
- a date for the next appointment, preferably within one week (Fig. 8.10, *see* page 150).

16 Record the outline plan, as envisaged at this stage.

Follow up visits

Allow 10-15 minutes, depending upon the anticipated nature of the consultation.

17 On the first follow up visit:

- build on the rapport already developed;
- check the patient's inhaler technique;
- answer any questions and gently revise and extend patient education as appropriate. It often helps to anticipate questions.

18 Follow up intervals will vary depending upon each patient's condition. Patients with seasonal asthma can have a planned consultation prior to the appearance of their symptoms to revise prophylactic strategy and treatment. A well motivated patient with well controlled asthma can be seen 2 or 3 times a year but the system must have sufficient flexibility to allow any patient to consult at any time. However well managed asthma is within the practice, emergencies will inevitably occur. Consequently, it is important that the GPs and nurses who are concerned with anticipatory care must not lose their expertise in handling acute exacerbations. The response must be prompt and vigorous.

Asthma Clinic
Bridge House Medical Centre
Scholars Lane
Stratford-upon-Avon CV37 6HE
Tel: 292201

REGULAR BRONCHODILATOR AND INHALED CORTICOSTEROID TREATMENT

Your asthma is such that to live a normal safe life you need to take a regular combination of inhaler treatments.

.... daily

.... daily

(after you have taken your ....)
plus extra .... if necessary

N.B. if you use a pressurised aerosol inhaler always leave at least 1 minute between puffs

*If in spite of this regular treatment you are persistently wheezy or coughing whether by day or night, or your peak flow rate stays below ...... then you should contact Mrs Barnes or Dr Pearson on the above telephone number.

*If you have been given a supply of prednisolone tablets (5 mg) for such occasions then immediately take **6** tablets with food BEFORE coming to see us.

Other instructions: ....

....

....

....

* Delete as applicable.

Figure 8.9 Treatment cards.

Asthma Clinic
Bridge House Medical Centre
Scholars Lane
Stratford-upon-Avon CV37 6HE
Tel: 292201

SODIUM CROMOGLYCATE (INTAL)

Sodium cromoglycate acts purely to PREVENT you having an asthma attack. It acts by stopping the release, in the lungs of some of the substances that cause asthma.

It is perfectly safe and is most effective in the prevention of allergic and exercise-induced asthma, especially in the young.

IT DOES NOT HAVE ANY EFFECT ON AN ASTHMATIC ATTACK WHICH HAS ALREADY STARTED.

If your asthma occurs in spite of using Intal, then you will require additional treatment.

Instructions ....

....

....

Asthma Clinic
Bridge House Medical Centre
Scholars Lane
Stratford-upon-Avon CV37 6HE
Tel: 292201

BRONCHODILATORS

Your bronchodilator, ... , works by relaxing the tight muscular coat around your small breathing tubes.

.... is a fast acting preventer and reverser of your asthma, and may be taken regularly as a prevention.

It is extremely safe and the dose which you are inhaling is very small. Your dosage is NOT limited by the safety of the drug - if you feel, however, that you need MORE than has been recommended, this suggests that you require an additional different treatment.

INHALED CORTICOSTEROIDS

Your inhaled corticosteroid .... works by reducing the swelling in your breathing tubes. .... is used when your bronchodilator alone is not wholly effective. It has no immediate action and needs to be taken as a REGULAR, long-term prevention in conjunction with your bronchodilator.

The dosage is very small as the active agent is inhaled directly into the lungs. Inevitably, some is deposited in the mouth and is swallowed, but at the doses recommended this has no detectable effect on the body. Soreness and white patches ('thrush') can occur at the back of the mouth but this can usually be avoided by having a drink after the inhalation.

It has been shown that twice daily inhalation is as effective as the same amount taken as four separate doses.

Occasionally, inhaled steroids may not be adequate and we may prescribe a course of corticosteroids by mouth.

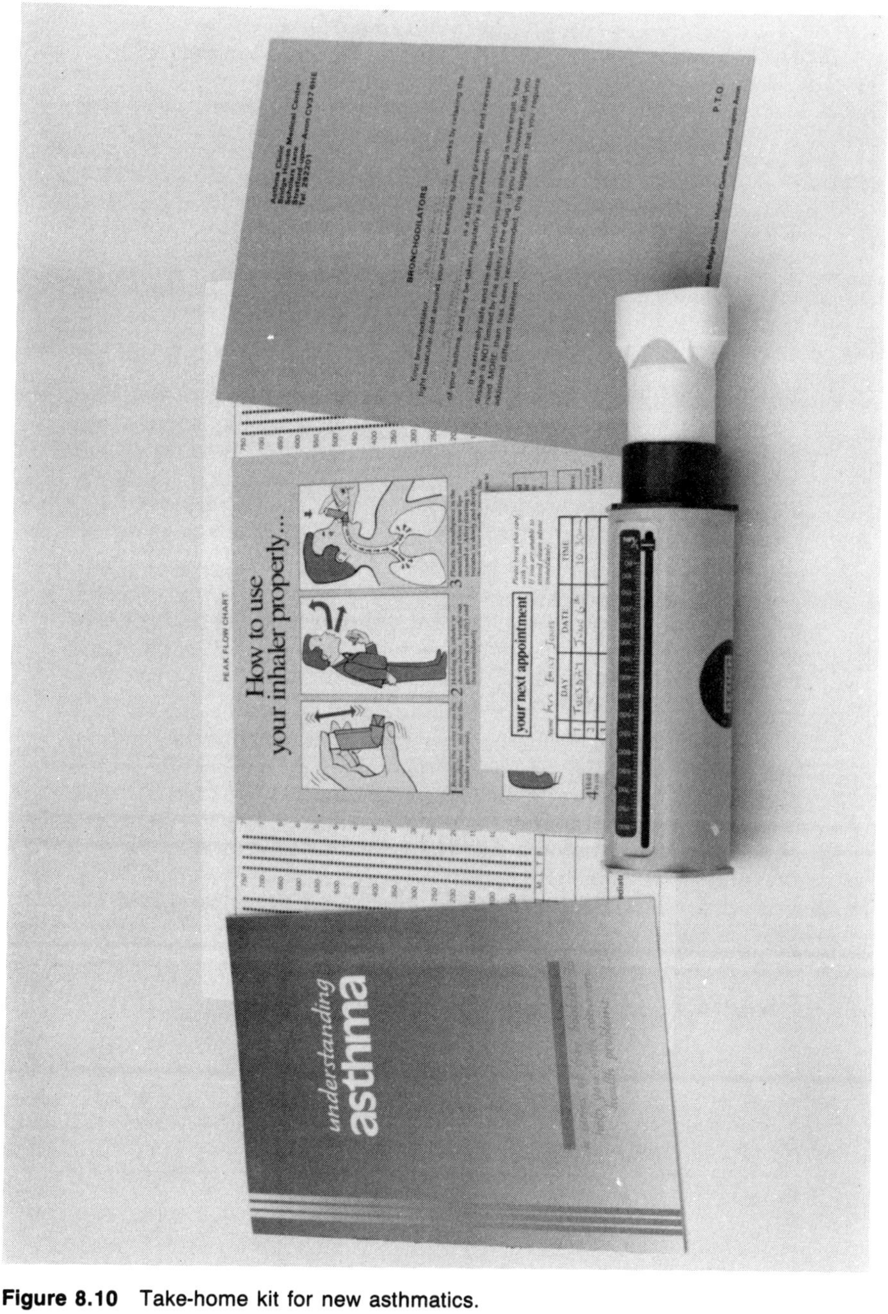

Figure 8.10 Take-home kit for new asthmatics.

19 Always check on symptoms and results of home monitoring, if appropriate.
20 Check on the patient's inhalation technique and compliance, especially if there is a history of recurring symptoms. Do not introduce new therapy or increase current therapy without ascertaining whether the patient is adhering to the planned regimen.
21 Perform reversibility tests when required, usually when the patient's asthma is inadequately controlled, to distinguish between bronchoconstriction and mucosal oedema.
22 Review and reassess therapy, discussing it with the patient *(consult the GP, if necessary).*
23 Revise the treatment card if necessary and maintain the momentum of the follow up by arranging another appointment.
24 Record the asthma attendance on the current record sheet so that reference can be made to the asthma card itself at a later date.

Useful points

- Ask patients to bring their own inhaler device with them either to check on inhalation technique or to perform a reversibility test.
- The asthma nurse must have free access to the patient's GP at the time of the consultation.
- Any nurse who has an extended role must not be asked to work beyond the limits of his or her training and ability.
- A specially trained nurse working in a general practice can act as a catalyst, but should not be allowed to work in a vacuum. Determining areas of responsibility taken by the GP and nurse requires teamwork and a common goal—there is no room for interprofessional competition.
- When a nurse is taking a major role in asthma care, the GP should conduct an annual review in order to maintain the GP – patient relationship and to form a planned part of the audit of that individual patient's asthma and of the practice's management of asthma.

Referral

In an ideal world there would be a simple hierarchical structure for asthma care. This would be along the lines which have evolved within the current National Health Service, with general practice being responsible for most asthma management and the thoracic medicine departments of hospitals providing further care and expertise for patients with more severe acute or chronic asthma.

It is important to examine why an asthma sufferer attends a hospital. Attendance may occur in two situations:

1 on referral by the patient's GP for an outpatient consultation;
2 in the event of an emergency.

Outpatient consultation

A patient is usually referred to a chest physician because:

1 there is some diagnostic uncertainty—the asthma might be symptomatic of a more complex disorder, such as polyarteritis nodosa, or the patient may have another diagnosis such as aspiration secondary to nocturnal oesophageal reflux;
2 after careful and logical treatment of the asthma, the patient's response to therapy is judged to be unsatisfactory.

Seeing such patients would be a sensible and productive use of a chest physician's time.

Unfortunately, some patients are referred when only bronchodilators have been prescribed. This would suggest that the GP has not progressed beyond bronchoconstriction to the consideration of mucosal problems as a significant element of asthma.

More often, sensible therapy has been prescribed but patient education, inhalation technique and compliance are woefully lacking so that the original plan has totally collapsed. This equates with a patient being seen in a chest clinic having stopped taking preventive therapy which he or she had only been using 'as required', because he or she thought that it was a 'stronger' drug but found it ineffective as used. The patient may have a bronchodilator aerosol inhaler which he or she cannot use properly so uses it far too frequently and without lasting benefit. Questioning of the patient reveals a series of misapprehensions and misconceptions.

Sometimes a referral may be made due to patient or family pressure. This may be because they feel that they need a specialist opinion and deem any GP to be second best. Usually they are seeking 'the cure', which they feel someone else must possess. Some of these patients or relatives may be happy to have their family doctor's approach vindicated in some circumstances, others may consult practitioners in various areas of alternative medicine.

There are occasions when patients have not been adequately diagnosed and treated, and in these cases the pressure from a patient or family to seek a further opinion is wholly justified. That this should occur is a sad reflection and the professions must do all in their power to make this a rare event.

If the time of chest physicians is taken up unnecessarily, then their expertise will not be available when it is required. Most asthmatics warrant effective treatment sooner rather than later and on occasion some patients will be admitted to the chest unit, rather than waiting for an outpatient visit, either at the suggestion of the chest physician or the GP, when it appears from the clinical circumstances that admission will be necessary.

At the other end of the referral system is the problem of disposal, or follow up. It is useful for the chest physician if the GP indicates his or her willingness to organize follow up when treatment is established, otherwise the hospital team may be reluctant to discharge the patient, especially when junior staff may not know the GP concerned. Any GP should be competent to manage asthma when guidelines have been drawn up by the chest physician. It is essential that all letters should be read and projected plans taken into account. Although a patient may have more intimate firsthand experience of asthma than the GP, it is unacceptable for a well informed patient to be better informed than the GP regarding asthma therapy. I have seen one old lady who had been prescribed prophylactic therapy, the rationale of which she understood, and who had the treatment stopped by her GP when she became asymptomatic 2 weeks later. She followed her doctor's advice and witnessed the predictable return of her symptoms!

Emergency hospital attendance

Although the aim of prophylactic therapy is to prevent severe exacerbations of asthma, there will be occasions when admission to a chest unit is necessary. The decline in function may have been rapid, over minutes or hours, or the result of an insidious deterioration over days or weeks, both of which can result in a worrying level of pulmonary function. The GP may have arranged the admission, having started immediate treatment at home, or the patient might be on the unit's self-referral list.

Problems are likely to arise in other less satisfactory situations. Some patients with exacerbations of asthma may be treated in accident and emergency departments. On such occasions, it is important that the attending doctor takes an appropriate history of what has led up to the problem. If this is part of a regular pattern, direct contact should be made with the patient's GP and the patient asked to attend for follow up. Failing this, the advice of the chest unit should be sought, but regular attendance in accident departments for nebulized bronchodilator therapy should be discouraged—there is no substitute for structured preventive therapy. A minority of GPs may actively or passively encourage their patients to attend hospital accident departments; equally, some patients may claim falsely that their GP was unavailable, perhaps because they have already defaulted from follow up and stopped regular therapy and they do not wish to be exposed.

Free access to children's wards may similarly encourage poor treatment, instead of concentrating on prophylactic therapy for this group of chronically or recurrently asthmatic children.

When patients are admitted to a chest unit with specially trained experienced staff, their treatment will be planned and consistent. If, however, patients enter a ward where the expertise lies in handling diabetic emergencies for example, there will be no in depth asthma care. Initial therapy may be given, but prophylactic care and follow up may be lacking. It has been shown that a considerably better, more predictable outcome is achieved when asthma patients are admitted to a chest unit, where all of the staff are skilled in assessment and treatment and, in particular, can recognize serious deterioration which might warrant assisted ventilation.

There is still considerable scope for closer liaison between hospitals and GPs. Communication needs to be more immediate; at present, it takes days or weeks before an effective report concerning an admission or a clinic visit reaches the GP. Conversely, the GP may have prescribed interim therapy about which the hospital team may be ignorant.

The National Asthma Campaign (previously the Asthma Society) has made some progress with the introduction of their asthma card for patients to carry with them (Fig. 8.11). It describes current therapy and advises on what action to take in the presence of any deterioration; it is not designed as a co-operation card. The latter has been used for many years for antenatal care and in some diabetic clinics, and the card is carried by the patient—to work, it needs to be filled in regularly by any attending doctor.

Nurse training

Special nurse training for asthma needs both theoretical instruction and practical experience. Naturally, the latter will need to be built upon after returning to one's working environment, with support from at least one GP.

Several excellent one-day courses have been sponsored by pharmaceutical companies, providing the theoretical background and practice with peak flow meters and inhalation devices. There are three-day courses designed to cover both needs, run for practice nurses (and other personnel) and their GPs, at the Asthma Training Centre, 22 Scholars Lane, Stratford upon Avon, Warwickshire CV37 6HE. Telephone: 0789 296974. Future courses will be certificated in order to provide a measure of proficiency. Such courses will include a distance learning package provided in conjunction with the Royal College of General Practitioners.

Audit

It is all too easy to be complacent and to assume that work could not be improved upon. Heavy workloads often allow little time for review and assessment. Deficiencies in care are caused partly by ignorance of advances and partly by a failure to apply current knowledge and therapies to patient care.

TREATMENT OF A SEVERE ATTACK

Suggestions for emergency doctor:

1. Gives salbutamol/terbutaline either via nebulizer 2.5 – 5mg or via larger spacer 8-16 puffs.
2. Give 40mg oral prednisolone if not already taken.
3. Give oxygen if available.
4. Injected therapy is sometimes necessary.

- slow s/c, i/m or i/v injection of:

  terbutaline)
  or) 0.25 - 0.5mg (0.5 - 1ml)
  salbutamol)

  or aminophylline 250mg slowly i/v
  (not s/c; not if on oral xanthines)

- 200mg hydrocortisone i/v

CARD CHECKED:

Date	Initials	Date	Initials

ASTHMA SOCIETY
ADULT'S ASTHMA CARD

Patient's Name ____________
Address ____________
____
____
Tel. No. ____________
General Practitioner ____________
Address: ____________
____
____
Tel. No: ____________
Consultant ____________
Hospital: ____________
Hospital Reference No.: ____________
Tel. No.: ____________

Always carry this card with you.

TREATMENT TO BE TAKEN REGULARLY

Treatment:	Dose: (No. of puffs or tablets)	No. of doses daily:

Don't forget your regular treatment.

RELIEF TREATMENT IF YOUR ASTHMA GETS WORSE

For sudden chest tightness, wheeze or breathlessness take:-

Name:	Dose and how taken:
1.	
2.	
3.	

If no relief or quickly worse:
- repeat relief treatment
- also take .... tablets of prednisolone*

And at the same time:
- contact your GP*
- or dial 999 for an ambulance*
- or go to .... Hospital

(*complete/delete as necessary)

Keep your inhalers handy at all times

IF YOU USE A PEAK FLOW METER FOLLOW THESE GUIDELINES

Expected Peak Flow ____________ l/min

Best Peak Flow ____________ l/min

If your Peak Expiratory Flow (PEF) sudddenly falls below ____________ use relief treatment in order listed.

If no relief or quickly worse again or if PEF at any time below ____________ take emergency action listed in the box on Page 3.

If your morning PEF is regularly below ____________ or you are waking at night with your asthma, see your Doctor.

You can obtain a Peak Flow Meter from the Asthma Society or through your doctor.

Figure 8.11 National Asthma Campaign (formerly Asthma Society) card.

If our current level of knowledge were applied fully, there would be a reduction in today's unnecessary morbidity and mortality. We need to bridge the gap between the world of pharmacological research and everyday medical practice. We must evolve patterns of care that suit both the providers and the recipients of that care; to do this, we must know what to provide, for whom, how and when. If a structured, logical plan for asthma management has been adopted, it is possible to provide the right care. The recipients should be identified by creating an asthma register of current and previous asthma sufferers. Management must be individually tailored as regards medication, dosage, timing and means of administration. The way in which care is provided will depend upon each practice's circumstances (staffing and geography, for example). The acceptability of the arrangements to patients ought to be tested, perhaps by an anonymous questionnaire. The time of day is important both from the viewpoint of the condition (diurnal variation) and of patient convenience.

We should ask simple questions relating to our individual practices—questions which can be answered fairly easily and whose answers can be compared with those of our peers.

1 Have all the asthmatic patients been identified?
2 Do you and your partners have a consistent approach to the diagnosis and management of asthma?
3 Does the individual history you take indicate trigger factors and the timing of symptoms, e.g. at night—the hallmark of bronchial hyperreactivity?
4 Is PEFR measured routinely during a consultation for asthma?
5 If so, are the results compared with the average values based on age, sex and height and with the patient's previous best?
6 Does the PEFR result influence treatment?
7 Are reversibility tests with bronchodilators or corticosteroids performed?
8 Do you use prophylactic drugs adequately?
9 Is there a clear record in the notes regarding currently *advised* therapy?
10 Is there a record of currently *taken* therapy?
11 Do you aim for maximum performance, bearing in mind that residual symptoms may equate with persistent bronchial wall inflammation and progression to irreversibility?
12 Do your patients understand their condition and its treatment?
13 Do your patients monitor their own PEFR?
14 Can you and do you demonstrate the different inhaler devices?
15 Do you encourage a system for follow up?

The patient audit means examining asthma status in order to test whether the maximum benefit is gained from the minimum amount of therapy.

It is possible to compare overall practice figures with those of individual GPs. The proportion of current asthma sufferers in the year in question can be identified and the level of prophylactic therapy in different age groups can be ascertained. It is no use being on the right medication if it cannot be used properly and so the types of devices are important. The number of patients who had their PEFR recorded and whether this altered their treatment was also checked. These are simple questions of relevance to our practice, the answers to which should encourage us to re-examine our practice of medicine.

9 The Intangibles of Asthma Care: Aspects of Patient, Family and Professional Psychology in Practice

'Nervous asthma!' – Resentment – Parental guilt – Problems of adolescence – Beware the unscrupulous – Patient education – What to do when

The diagnosis of asthma still has a stigma attached to it, and in some quarters is still associated with fear. Many asthmatics are still shouldering the unfair burden of being labelled as suffering from 'nervous asthma'—a condition of the psyche rather than of the lungs. This dates from an era of therapeutic impotence, when non-pharmacological remedies were tried in many patients with severe chronic asthma. The implication of the label was that the condition was largely the fault of the patient, not his or her genes or environment. It is easy to understand why some asthmatics can become very anxious and apprehensive if they are severely breathless as the result of asthma. However, no pattern of psychological disturbance has been found in asthma sufferers. It is hardly remarkable that the control of asthma is accompanied by considerable relief on the patient's part. It is most rewarding to attend patients who have better lung function now than they had when desperately attending for hypnotherapy over twenty years ago, despite the effects of ageing. It is important to be honest about the diagnosis because this is the only way to achieve effective treatment. However, the impact of the diagnosis on the condition itself should not be underestimated.

The diagnosis of asthma in children is likely to give rise to considerable parental guilt which may manifest itself in various ways—such as aggression towards the child or conflict between the parents, particularly if one is held to be responsible. Close relatives may have their own memories of asthma, from days when little therapy was available and they may relive stories of the doctor sitting with them at night, injecting subcutaneous adrenaline. The 'nervous asthma' title will be bandied about, perhaps associated with the image of someone who is very restricted in their physical activities. As with other potentially intrusive chronic disorders, which are also treatable, such as insulin-dependent diabetes mellitus, the patient may so resent the diagnosis and the fact that it has happened to him or her, that he or she may fail to accept it and come to terms with it, so that proper self-treatment becomes impossible. Psychological problems are usually the result of asthma, rather than its cause.

How does the condition itself affect the patient and his or her family? The patient's life may be quite disrupted, with tiredness due to disturbed nights. The inability to breathe easily may be frightening and lead to hyperventilation and its associated problems. Apart from physical restrictions, chronic ill health can lead to the loss of time from work or school and severely affect the patient's social life. This pattern in early life can lead to lowered expectations and may restrict the number of occupations which can be followed.

Whether due to guilt or total lack of insight, a family's reactions may be directed against the sufferer, perhaps because of sleepless nights or the disruption of family plans when the asthma is a problem. A parent may belittle or reject his or her child, making light of the diagnosis and treating the child as if he or she is deficient in some way. On the other hand, the guilt or family concern may result in the patient being smothered and over protected—never allowed to go far for fear of an attack. A child in particular, but adults too, will need understanding and encouragement. Family support should be positive. This requires members of the family to be informed and educated about asthma and its management. This may suggest the need for a widening of lay education on this as on other medical and health matters.

Adolescence presents its own problems and conflicts even without the introduction of a disorder such as asthma. Most well adjusted adolescents will cope well with managing their asthma, the only difference in their life being their regular medication. Some asthmatics may use their asthma to manipulate those close to them, whether they are parents, friends or teachers. Asthma which is well treated is more difficult to precipitate at will, and this may lead to the neglect of therapy in order to produce a state of bronchial hyperreactivity which will allow rapid bronchoconstriction to occur, perhaps induced by deliberate coughing or hyperventilation. Complex or disturbed family backgrounds may encourage this type of behaviour pattern, when it may appear that affection has to be fought for. Fortunately, the advent of modern treatment has transformed the lives of most asthmatics, but for those with severe social and psychological problems the threat to refuse to take treatment may be a powerful weapon, which may serve to magnify the guilt felt by many parents.

Patients with chronic disorders are vulnerable. We are not able to offer cures but can provide long term treatment which will effectively suppress the pathological process. Some patients or their relatives will set off in pursuit of the elusive cure and will explore all avenues. There have always been fringe operators, but recently many new forms of alternative medicine have been developed and pressed upon a naïve public. Most have no tested, rational or scientific basis but they will always find someone looking for a cure. Unfortunately, while the practices of doctors and nurses are governed by licensing bodies, no such regulation occurs in the alternative spheres. While some asthmatics may come to no harm, others may suffer, especially if advised to stop taking their medical treatment.

One thing that alternative practitioners may offer is time—the time to discuss many problems, some associated with asthma but others which may be important to them and perhaps indirectly concerned with their asthma. Doctors and nurses must develop a good therapeutic relationship with their patients whereby patients feel able to discuss these problems with them. We need also to make more time if possible. Equally, we have to recognize that a poor relationship with the patient may result in an unsympathetic attitude to his or her problems. It is always important that we as professionals are aware of our own feelings towards the patient, whether they are positive or negative.

The patient: patient education

In order to manage asthma in its broadest sense, we must develop empathy with the patient. This does not mean that we should be sympathetic and feel sorry for the patient as these are sentiments which may have a negative effect. If nurses are to adapt their traditional role of comforter and hand holder to assist in the active management of dynamic disorders they must examine and analyse good doctor – patient relationships which are closer to the new role that the nurse must adopt. In order to be of assistance in explaining the diagnosis, its implications and the projected treatment plan we must have insight into the individual patient's situation. It is unsafe to assume knowledge, even in patients who may be health professionals. The implications of asthma or its treatment will vary according to age, sex, intelligence, occupation and family environment.

If we start with a simple explanation of the mechanisms of asthma, preferably illustrated by a drawing, we can then progress to explaining the logic of therapy and its adjustment. As described earlier, the aim of management is a patient who can manage his or her own asthma with help and guidance. Parents must accept ultimate responsibility for their children, and supervision must be sensitive and not overbearing, even though there may be a high level of concern.

Asthma in school causes concern, particularly if children have asthma attacks. Asthmatic children may not be allowed to do games or to take inhalers to school. Health professionals have a role to play in educating teachers and providing notes for children to take to school.

At least 50% of current asthmatics would benefit from regular preventive therapy. The average hypertensive patient will take hypotensive medication as directed, probably because hypertension is usually asymptomatic and there is no cue to stop therapy. However, asthma is a symptomatic condition and many patients' instincts will tell them to stop their treatment after their symptoms have been suppressed, even if they have had the rationale of therapy explained to them.

For some patients, the return of symptoms after the cessation of therapy is a valuable educational exercise. Unfortunately, some patients simply reduce or stop prophylactic therapy, consuming ever increasing amounts of bronchodilators. While I advocate and provide written instructions for patients, I appreciate that some patients will lose the instructions and explanations, just as they forget their verbal counterparts. This makes follow up all the more important if we wish to keep people well—educational input must be reinforced verbally and with leaflets and videos.

A patient must be equipped with the knowledge to allow him or her to take appropriate action in the event of deterioration in his or her asthma. This requires knowledge of the actions of their drugs and ideally possession of some means of self monitoring such as a mini peak flow meter. Some patients on regular prophylactic therapy will need to have a supply of corticosteroids at home in order to embark upon a course if the asthma deteriorates to a pre-determined level.

It has been our practice to attempt to tailor each individual's therapy, with instructions on how to respond to deteriorating asthma, as judged by symptoms and by PEFR measurements. The Southampton group (Beasley et al.) have tried a similar but generalized scheme for their patients who are on regular inhaled corticosteroids using daily morning PEFR measurements. They start by attaining optimal function in each patient, when their PEFR is taken to be their 'potential normal value'. Above 70% of this value they continue their twice daily regimen of inhaled beta$_2$-agonist and inhaled corticosteroid, but if the morning PEFR is between 50 and 70%, they double the inhaled corticosteroid intake, taking it 4 times daily rather than twice, until the PEFR returns to baseline, then continuing at this dosage for the same number of days before reducing to the usual maintenance dosage. Below 50%, oral prednisolone is commenced, in a dosage of 40 mg daily, to obtain a return to baseline before reducing to 20 mg daily for the same length of time, then stopping. As in our scheme, the patient is advised to contact their GP at the same time. With a PEFR as low as an arbitrary 150 – 200 l/min the patient is instructed to call their GP urgently or, failing that, the ambulance service and to go directly to the respiratory unit. There is a group whose asthma is too brittle to adhere to this regimen, sometimes because of the asthma itself, but occasionally because of inconsistently taken prophylactic therapy. In these cases, it is necessary to start on oral prednisolone as soon as the airflow limitation becomes refractory to the inhaled $beta_2$-agonist or the PEFR falls to a preset level, which may be above 70% optimum on occasion. These patients will deteriorate relentlessly if they do not commence oral prednisolone at once.

The means of administration must be checked, so that dosages are correct and appropriate and that technique is consistent. The use of inhaled steroids or systemic steroids must be explained and the patient must realize that they are safe in taking controlled doses of corticosteroids under supervision. The vision of real or imaginary side effects must be dispelled or put into perspective.

Until recently, the most common causes of poor treatment of asthma were that the wrong diagnosis had been made, or that in the presence of the correct diagnosis, inappropriate therapy had been prescribed. With the new awareness of asthma, the correct treatment might be prescribed, but an inadequate dosage may have been advised, or the patient may be taking it inconsistently. Remember that patients will usually avoid lying to their doctor or nurse but may be able to avoid telling the absolute truth if a question has been worded loosely. Direct questions on compliance must be posed. They provide the means whereby the patient can be totally honest, without loss of face: 'How many times a week do you forget your regular preventive therapy, bearing in mind how busy you are?'

During consultations, many questions will arise which should be answered honestly and fully. Usually these questions will be sensible and understandable, but sometimes they will serve to illustrate the lack of understanding among the general public.

Questions

- Are inhalers addictive?
- Aren't puffers dangerous?
- If I use it (any therapeutic agent) now, will it work when I really need it?
- Steroids have serious side effects, don't they?
- Do I have an infection if my phlegm is discoloured?
- Will asthma/asthma treatment stunt his/her growth?
- The teacher won't let him/her take his/her inhaler to school. What shall I do?
- How can we find out what he/she is allergic to?
- Is he/she allowed to play any games?
- What jobs can I do with asthma?
- Will I pass it on to my children?
- Will he/she grow out of it?
- It won't hurt if his father and I smoke, will it?
- Should we move to the south coast (east coast or west coast)?
- Are my inhalers allowed if I run competitively?

A very good selection of leaflets and educational videos, covering most aspects of asthma, are available from various sources, particularly the National Asthma Campaign and pharmaceutical companies. Most of the informational material is non-promotional but it is advisable to check before giving it to patients or relatives (Fig. 9.1). Education is a continuous process.

Addresses

British Lung Foundation
Kingsmead House, 250 Kings Road, London SW3 5UE.
Telephone 01 376 5735
Allen and Hanburys Ltd
Greenford, Middlesex UB6 0HE
Telephone 01 422 4225
Astra Pharmaceuticals Ltd
Home Park Estate, Kings Langley, Herts WD4 8DH
Telephone 09277 66191
Boehringer Ingelheim Ltd
Ellesfield Avenue, Bracknell, Berks RG12 4YS
Telephone 0344 424600
Fisons PLC
Pharmaceutical Divn., 12 Derby Road, Loughborough, Leics LE11 0BB
Telephone 0509 611001
3M Riker
Morley Street, Loughborough, Leics LE11 1EP
Telephone 0509 611611
Napp Laboratories
The Science Park, Cambridge CB4 4GW
Telephone 0223 358888
National Asthma Campaign (previously the Asthma Society and Friends of the Asthma Research Council)
300 Upper Street, London N1 2XX. Telephone 01 226 2260
Pfizer Ltd
Sandwich, Kent CT13 9NJ
Telephone 0304 616161

Patients are able to purchase mini Wright peak flow meters at discount prices by application to the National Asthma Campaign, Allen and Hanburys and Fisons. The patient will need help from his or her doctor and practice nurse in how best to use the peak flow meter to assist in the management of his or her own asthma—it is no use the patient accumulating meaningless pages of peak flow values—measurements must have a purpose.

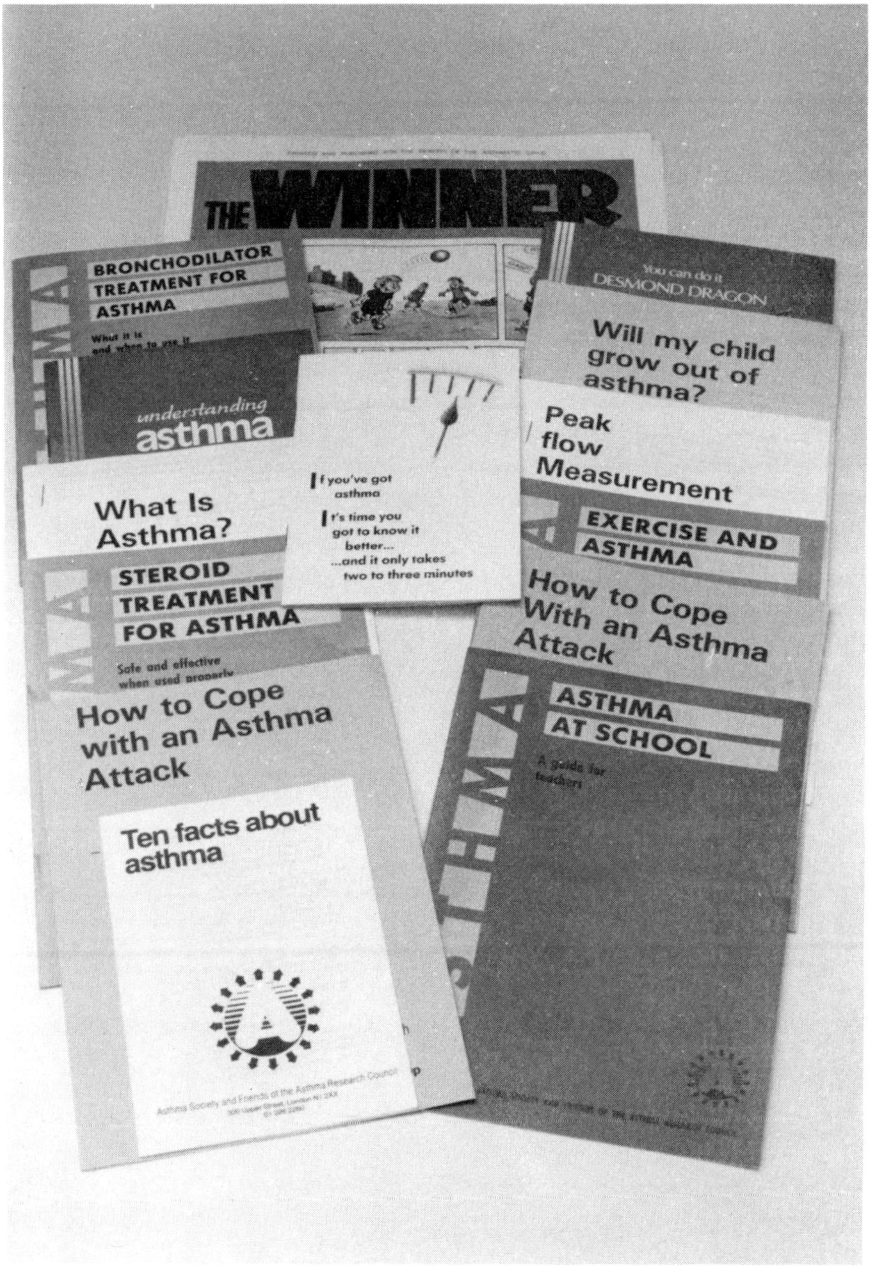

Figure 9.1. Educational leaflets for patients.

10 The Future

WE are in a fortunate position – the inhaled drugs at our disposal are safe and effective when applied appropriately. Logical forethought should allow the experienced professional to match therapy to patients. Our greatest problem is not that many asthmatics are untreatable using current therapies, but that many asthmatics are not treated or are unsuccessfully using the wrong treatments. Further improvements in the provision of correct care must be the foundation for better services to asthma sufferers. It is true to say that those who have been well trained, can flexibly assess an individual's asthma problems and sensitively apply their own expertise, will be able to manage most asthma very successfully – as long as it is done well it is irrelevant who provides the care.

Selected nurses, who feel that they are confident to apply specialist knowledge, are in a privileged position. We must remember that they do not need to 'unlearn' the practices of the 1960's and early 1970's – overuse of bronchodilators and antibiotics. Newly trained 'asthma nurses' and tomorrow's doctors should start out with virgin minds and it is our responsibility to equip them with the appropriate information on pathophysiology and patient behaviour to enable them to treat asthma properly from the start.

While most asthma is potentially controllable, there are some patients whose asthma defies our efforts. Some patients will display morning dips in spite of maximal current bronchial anti-inflammatory therapy. Others show a capacity consistently to consume beta$_2$-agonists at a fast rate so that their normally reasonable duration of action is considerable shortened.

Two types of development may help such patients. In the near future we are likely to see two new inhaled long acting selective beta$_2$-agonist bronchodilators, formoterol and salmeterol. Formoterol has a speed of onset which is as fast as salbutamol but its effect is still very significant 12 hours after inhalation, while most of the effect of salbutamol has gone by 4 hours. In a dosage of 12 μg per puff (2 puffs, twice daily) formoterol has already proved more popular than currently available beta$_2$-agonists in clinical trials. It is to be hoped that it will prove to be useful in treating nocturnal asthma that is resistant to inhaled anti-inflammatory therapy. Salmeterol was developed to make use of the known efficacy of the current beta$_2$-agonists by altering the 'tail' of the pre-existing molecule to make it more adherent to the cell membrane in order to extend its duration of action. Its onset of action is slower than that of salbutamol and its place may be in providing prolonged rather than rapid bronchodilatation. Ultimate bronchodilatation resulting from 50 μg of salmeterol is equivalent to that following the inhalation of 200 μg of salbutamol. An interesting point, to confirm that it is receptor activity which is all important, is that the plasma half lives of salbutamol and salmeterol are similar but the durations of clinical action are very different. We await with interest these twice daily inhaled $beta_2$-agonists. While their effects on bronchial smooth muscle relaxation, inhibition of release of preformed mast cell mediators and increasing mucociliary transport are known, we must await long term clinical studies to assess whether they have any additional anti-inflammatory effect at clinical dosage.

Agents which are designed for their anti-inflammatory action will undoubtedly appear, such as PAF-antagonists (platelet-activating factor *see* Fig. 2.7, page 22). It has been known for some time that substances such as gingkolides from the Chinese gingko tree have PAF-antagonizing effects and drugs which share this action are being developed. Such developments are exciting but we must await clinical trials before we comment further. Guarded optimism might be appropriate but so many previous attempts to curb the effects of particular cells and mediators have not met with great success. However, PAF does appear to play a central, ubiquitous role in bronchial inflammation and hyperreactivity and the development of such agents may help some patients whose asthma resists our efforts at present.

An exciting time ahead, both in the application of current drugs and the introduction of new ones – what is certain is that there appears to be *no* panacea on the horizon!

Useful reading

Clark, T. J. H. & Godfrey, S. (1983) Asthma. Chapman and Hall, London.

Clark, T. J. H. & Rees, J. (1985) Practical management of asthma. Martin Dunitz, London.

Woodcock, A. A. & Partridge, M. R. (1986) Respiratory Handbook. Boehringer Ingelheim.

Lee, D. A., Winslow, N. R., Speight, A. W. P. & Hey, E.N. (1983) Prevalence and spectrum of asthma in childhood. *British Medical Journal,* **286:** 1256 – 1258.

Speight, A. W. P., Lee, D. A. & Hey, E. N. (1983) Underdiagnosis and undertreatment of asthma in childhood. *British Medical Journal,* **286:** 1253 – 1256.

British Thoracic Association (1982) Death from asthma in two regions of England. *British Medical Journal,* **285:** 1251 – 1255.
Steventon, R. D. & Wilson, R. S. E. (1986) A guide to apparatus for home nebulizer therapy. Allen and Hanburys.
Beasley, R., Cushley, M. & Holgate, S. T. (1989) A self management plan in the treatment of adult asthma. *Thorax*, **44:** 200 – 204.

Appendix 1

Relative monthly prescribing cost (as at May 1989)

Over £20.00		*Dose*	*Number of doses*
Terbutaline	Bricanyl Respules	5 mg	20
Salbutamol	Ventolin Nebules	2.5 mg	20
Salbutamol	Ventolin Nebules	5 mg	20
Ipratropium	Atrovent solution	500 μg	10
Beclomethasone	Becodisks	200 μg	112
Beclomethasone	Becodisks	400 μg	56
Ketotifen	Zaditen tabs	1 mg	60
£15.00 – £19.99			
Nedocromil sodium	Tilade inhaler	2 mg	112
Beclomethasone	Becotide Rotacaps	200 μg	100
Beclomethasone	Becotide Rotacaps	400 μg	100
£10.00 – £14.99			
Sodium cromoglycate	Intal inhaler	5 mg	112
Salbutamol	Aerolin Autohaler	100 μg	200
Salbutamol	Ventolin Rotacaps	400 μg	100
Salbutamol	Ventodisks	400 μg	112
Salbutamol	Volmax tabs	8 mg	56
Terbutaline	Bricanyl Turbohaler	500 μg	200
Sodium cromoglycate	Intal Spincaps	20 mg	112
Beclomethasone	Becloforte inhaler	250 μg	200
Beclomethasone	Becodisks	100 μg	112
Under £10.00			
Salbutamol	Cobutolin	100 μg	200
Salbutamol	Salbulin	100 μg	200
Salbutamol	Salbuvent	100 μg	200
Salbutamol	Ventolin	100 μg	200
Salbutamol	Ventolin Rotacaps	200 μg	100
Salbutamol	Ventodisks	200 μg	112
Terbutaline	Bricanyl inhaler	250 μg	400
Ipratropium	Atrovent inhaler	18 μg	200
Ipratropium	Atrovent forte inhaler	36 μg	200

		Dose	*Number of doses*
Fenoterol	Berotec inhaler	200 μg	200
Reproterol	Bronchodil inhaler	500 μg	400
Pirbuterol	Exirel inhaler	200 μg	200
Beclomethasone	Becotide 50 inhaler	50 μg	200
Beclomethasone	Becotide 100 inhaler	100 μg	200
Beclomethasone	Becotide Rotacaps	100 μg	100
Budesonide	Pulmicort	200 μg	200
Budesonide	Pulmicort LS	50 μg	200
Theophylline	Slophyllin caps	60 mg	100
Theophylline	Slophyllin caps	125 mg	100
Theophylline	Slophyllin caps	250 mg	100
Theophylline	Uniphyllin continus	300 mg	56
Theophylline	Uniphyllin continus	400 mg	56

Hay fever treatments – under £15.00

Acrivastine	Semprex cap	8 mg	100
Astemizole	Hismanal tabs	10 mg	30
Cetirizine	Zirtek	10 mg	30
Terfenadine	Triludan	60 mg	60
Terfenadine	Triludan forte	120 mg	30

Eye drops – under £10.00

Sodium cromoglycate	Opticrom aqueous	2%	13.5 ml

Nasal treatments – under £10.00

Sodium cromoglycate	Rynacrom spray	2%	26 ml
Beclomethasone	Beconase aerosol	50 μg	200
Beclomethasone	Beconase aqueous	50 μg	200
Budesonide	Rhinocort aerosol	50 μg	200
Flunisolide	Syntaris aqueous	25 μg	24 ml

Appendix 2

Normal peak flow readings in adults

Gregg I, Nunn AJ. Br Med J 1973;3:282

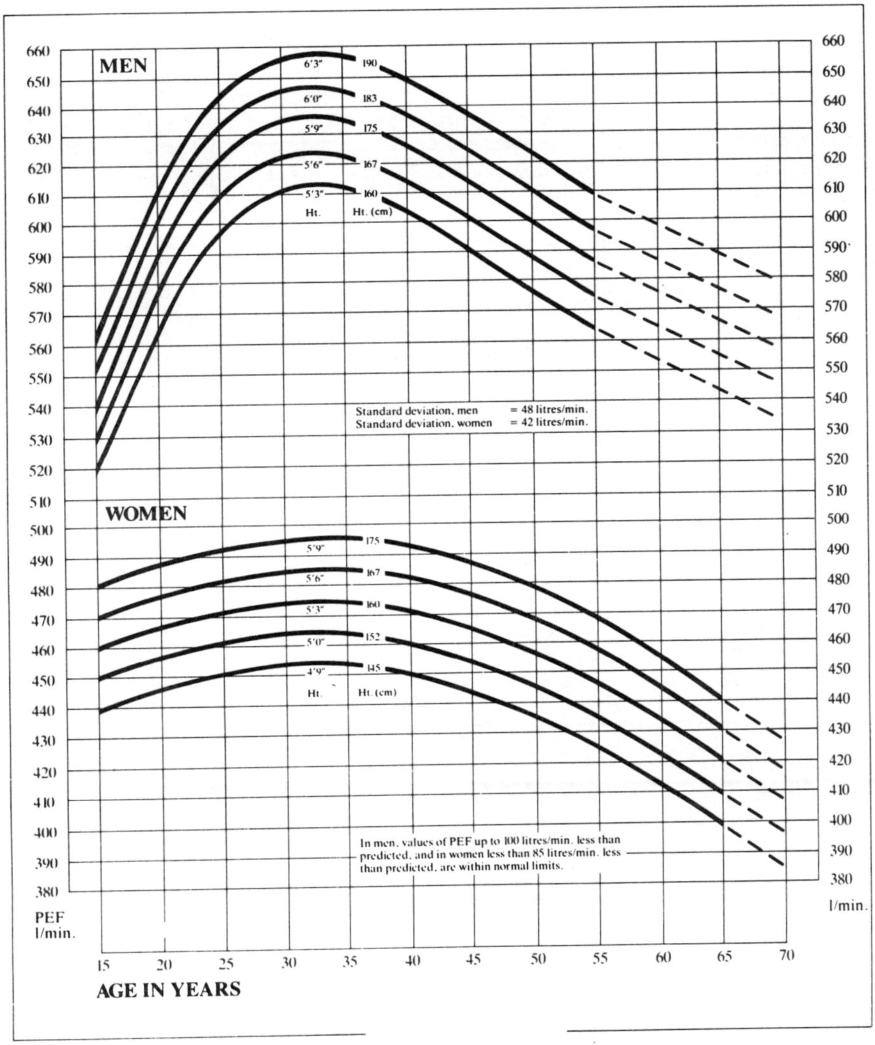

Normal peak flow readings for children aged 5 to 18 years

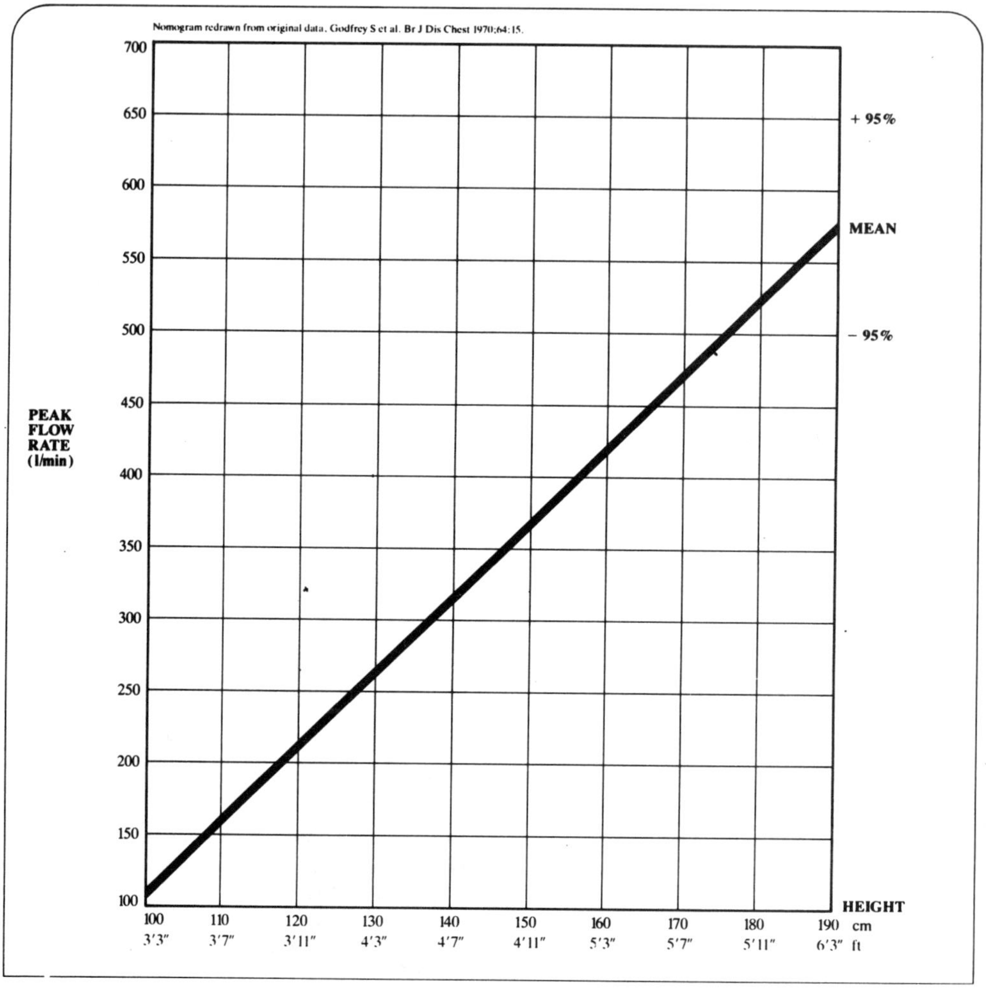

This nomogram results from tests carried out by Prof. S. Godfrey and his colleagues on a sample of 382 normal boys and girls aged 5 to 18 years. Each child blew five times into a standard Wright Peak Flow Meter and the highest reading was accepted in each case. All measurements were completed within a 6-week period. The outer lines of the graph indicated that the results of 95% of the children fell within these boundaries.

Index

absenteeism 26
ACTH 80
  see also corticosteroids, systemic
adolescence 160
  patterns of presentation in 39
  treatment 123–4
    acute 126–8
    preventive 123–6, 128
adrenaline 75
  aerosols 75–6
adulthood
  patterns of presentation in 39
  treatment 129
    acute 131–3
    preventive 129–31, 133
Aerolin Autohaler 94
aerosols, metered-dose 92, 94, 99
  in adolescence and late childhood 124
  compatibility with expansion chambers 95
  problems with 75–6
age patterns 38–9
allergic bronchopulmonary aspergillosis 49
allergic conjunctivitis 13, 134
allergic reactions 12
  to ingested allergens 31
  to inhaled particles 30–1
  as trigger factors 29–30
  see also atopy
$alpha_1$ antitrypsin deficiency 45
alpha-receptors 76–7
alternative therapies 32, 160–1
alveoli 3–4
alveolitis 45
aminophylline, intravenous 100, 127, 132
anatomical dead space 7
angina pectoris 79
angioneurotic oedema 31
annual review 151
antibiotic therapy 29, 120, 133
anticholinergics 33, 58, 79–80
  in adult life 130
  in drug combinations 89
  in infancy 118
  reversibility test 72
anticipatory care 139
antihistamines 134
arachidonic acid 19
Aspergillus, allergic reactions to 49
aspirin sensitivity 11, 34
asthma card 155
Asthma Society Training Centre 154
atelectasis 48
atopy 11, 12–14
  inheritance 30
audit 113, 154, 156–7

barbiturates 89
basophil chemotactic factor 19
beclomethasone dipropionate 82–3
  in drug combinations 89
  dry powder delivery 96
  in hay fever/rhinitis 134
  see also corticosteroids, inhaled
$beta_2$-agonists 76–8
  administration 78–9, 100
  in adolescence 123, 124
  in adult life 130
  dosage 78–9
  in drug combinations 89
  future developments 162–3
  in infancy 118
  reversibility test 72
  side effects 79
  sustained-release 131
  syrup formulations 90, 118
beta-blockers 4
  as trigger factors 34
betamethasone 83
  see also corticosteroids, inhaled
beta-receptors 76
blood-flow, pulmonary 6
breathing 1
  control of 6–7
breathlessness 14, 37
  in infancy 38
bronchi
  anatomy and physiology 2–5
  pathological features 14–15
bronchial hyperreactivity 15, 19, 21
  treatment principles 110, 111–13
  after viral infection 28
bronchial obstruction, differential diagnosis 40
bronchiectasis 1
  differential diagnosis 41–2
bronchioles
  anatomy and physiology 2–5
  pathological features 14–15

bronchiolitis 30–1
  differential diagnosis 40
bronchitis
  acute 40
  misdiagnosis 39
  'wheezy' 38
bronchoconstriction 14, 15, 16, 19, 22
  treatment principles 110, 114
bronchodilators 76–80
  see also specific types
budesonide 83–4
  in hay fever/rhinitis 134
  see also corticosteroids, inhaled

candidiasis, oral 84, 94, 123
cardiovascular system, examination 104
care
  deficiencies in 101–2
  organization of 138–41
case histories 135–8
catecholamines 4
chest
  deformity 50
  silent 53
  X-ray 104
childhood
  early *see* infancy
  patterns of presentation in 38–9
  treatment 124–5
    acute 126–8
    preventive 123–4, 128
cigarettes *see* tobacco smoking
classification 10–12
clinic 142–3
  organization 143, 145–6, 151
clinic record card 143, 144
clinical review 121
cold air as trigger factor 33
compliance in adolescence 126
complications
  acute 47–51
  chronic 49–51
corticosteroids 80–1
  in drug combinations 89
  effects on growth 50, 82, 123
  inhaled 82–4
    in adolescence 125
    in adult life 130–1
    in infancy 119
  injections 100, 134
  reversibility test 72
  systemic 81–2, 110, 114
    in adolescence 126, 127
    in adult life 131, 132–3
    in infancy 120, 121, 122
  topical 134, 135
cough 14, 37
  in infancy 38, 115

croup, differential diagnosis 43
cyclo-oxygenase pathway 19
cystic fibrosis, differential
  diagnosis 43–4

definitions 9–10
'degree of paradox' 127
Dermatophagoides pteronyssimus 30
desensitization 31
diagnosis 102–4, 107, 110
diagnostic tests 71–3
differential diagnosis 40–6
Diskhaler 96
drugs, anti-asthma 75–90
  combinations 89
  delivery systems 91–100, 114
  trade names 90
  see also specific types and drugs
dry powder inhalers 95–6, 98
  in adolescence 123–4
  in childhood 118
  in old age 130
'dual response' 16, 18, 19–21
Duovent 89
dyspepsia 133
dyspnoea 14, 37
  in infancy 38
dysrhythmias 79

'early asthmatic response' 16, 18, 19–21
eczema 11, 135
emotion as trigger factor 33
emphysema 44–5
eosinophil chemotactic factor 19
ephedrine 89
epidemiology 25
epiglottitis 43
'ethnic corrections' in lung function
  tests 54
ethnic factors in prevalence 25
exercise-induced asthma 10, 32–3, 129
  diagnostic test 71
exercise test 71
expansion chambers 94–5, 118
external respiration 1
extrinsic asthma 10, 11

family, effects of asthma on 159–60
fenoterol 77
  in drug combinations 89
  see also beta$_2$-agonists
FEV_1 54, 60, 66
  paradoxical rise 60, 65
flow chart, diagnostic 104, 108–9
flow-volume measurements 54, 67, 70
flunisolide 134
follow up 140–1, 142, 143, 146, 151
  after an outpatient visit 153

food additives 31–2
forced expiratory volume in one
  second 54, 60, 66
  paradoxical rise 60, 65
forced vital capacity 60, 64, 66, 67, 70
formoterol 167
functional residual capacity 60
fungal spores 30
future developments 167–8
FVC 60, 64, 66, 67, 70

gaseous exchange 1, 4
gastro-oesophageal reflux as trigger
  factor 35
general practice, care within 139
gingkolides 168
goblet cells 2, 3
  innervation 4
growth
  effect of asthma on 26, 50
  effect of corticosteroids on 50,
    82, 123
  as indicator of control 123

Haemophilus influenzae infection 43
  as trigger factor 29
hay fever 11, 134
  desensitization 31
histamine 19
history-taking 103–4
hoarseness due to inhaled steroids 84
hospital admission
  in adolescence and late childhood 127
  in adult life 132
  emergency 153–4
  in infancy and early childhood
    121
  self-referral 139
house dust mite 30
hydrocortisone 100, 132
hypersensitivity reactions 12
  Type I 12–14, 19–21
hyperventilation
  differential diagnosis 42–3
  as trigger factor 33
hyposensitization 31

ibuprofen sensitivity 34
IgE 12–14
immotile cilia syndromes 42
immunodeficiency 42
immunoglobulin E 12–14
industrial substances recognized for
  compensation 12
infancy
  assessment of intermittent
    symptoms 73
  drug therapy delivery 96, 98
  patterns of presentation 38
  treatment 115
    acute 120–22
    preventive 118–20
information sources 164
ingested allergens 31–2
inhaled allergens 30–1
inhaled foreign bodies, differential
  diagnosis 41
inhaled therapy 91–100
  see also specific drugs and systems
initial assessment 145–6
injections 100
inspiratory stridor, differential
  diagnosis 43
Intal *see* sodium cromoglycate
intrinsic asthma 10, 11
ipratropium bromide 33, 58, 79–80
  in adult life 130
  in drug combinations 89
  in infancy 118
  reversibility test 72
irreversible airflow limitation
  differential diagnosis 44–5
  due to asthma 53
irritant receptors 4
isoprenaline 77
  aerosols, problems with 75–6
  in drug combinations 85, 89

ketotifen 88–9

'late asthmatic response' 16, 18, 19–21
laughter as trigger factor 33
lipomodulin 80–1
lipoxygenase pathway 19
lower respiratory tract, anatomy and
  physiology 2–5
lung function tests 53–73
lung volumes 67
lungs 2–3
  reserve capacity 7
  sensory receptors 4

macrocortin 80–1
manipulation of symptoms 160
mast cells 12, 13–14
  degranulation 19–20, 32
mediastinal emphysema 48, 49, 104, 105
medulla oblongata 6
medullary chemoreceptors 6
membrane-derived mediators 19, 33
menstrual factors 35
methylxanthines *see* theophylline
mini Wright peak flow meter 55, 164
morbidity 25–7
'morning dip' 14, 25, 58, 59
mortality 26, 27, 131

mucosal inflammation 2, 14, 15, 19, 20, 22
  treatment principles 113–14
mucus
  plugging 48
  secretion 14, 15, 19, 37–8

nasal polyps 11
Nebuhaler 95, 96, 98
  in infancy 115–16
nebulizers 98–9
  in infancy 118
nedocromil sodium 85–6
  in adolescence 125
  in adult life 131
neoplasms, differential diagnosis 41
'nervous asthma' 159
neuropeptides 4
neutrophil chemotactic factor 19, 32
nocturnal disturbance 25–6, 115
non-steroidal anti-inflammatory drugs (NSAIDs), sensitivity to 34
nurse
  role in care 141–2, 151
  training 154

obesity 129
occupational asthma 10, 11–12
oral therapy 91–2
oropharynx 1
  candidiasis due to inhaled corticosteroids 84, 94, 123
outpatient consultation 152–3
oxygen therapy 132

PAF *see* platelet-activating factor
parenchymal lung disease, differential diagnosis 45–6
parental guilt 160
pathophysiology 14–21
patient education 141, 161–4
patient register 143, 145
peak expiratory flow rate (PEFR) 54, 55–7
  in childhood 119
  home monitoring 57–8, 111
  use in tailoring treatment 162–3
peptic ulceration 133
perennial rhinitis 11, 13, 134
pets, allergic reations to 31
physical examination 104
platelet-activating factor (PAF) 21
  antagonists 168
pneumotachograph 70
pneumothorax 47–8, 127
Pocket Spirometer 69, 70
pollen 30
polyarteritis nodosa 45

posture, during lung function tests 54
practitioners, non-medically qualified 32, 160–1
prednisolone 79
  dosage 80
  see also corticosteroids, systemic
prednisone 81
pregnancy 35
prevalence 21, 23–5
prophylactic therapy 110, 111–13
  in adolescence and late childhood 124–6, 128
  in adult life 129–31, 133
  in exercise-induced asthma 32–3
  importance of 139–40
  in infancy and early childhood 118–21, 122
  in pregnancy 35
  see also specific agents
provocation tests 73
psychological factors in asthma 33, 159–61
puberty, delayed 26, 50
pulmonary oedema, differential diagnosis 44
pulsus paradoxus 127

quality of life 160

referral 151–2
REM sleep, interference with 25, 50
reproterol 77
  see also beta$_2$-agonists
residual volume 66, 67
respiration 1
respiratory syncytial virus 30, 40
respiratory system, anatomy and physiology 1–5
reversibility tests 72–3
rhinoviruses as trigger factors 28–9
rimiterol 79
Rondo 95
Rotahaler 96
RSV 30, 40

salbutamol 77
  dosage 78–9
  in drug combinations 89
  dry powder delivery 95–6
  reversibility test 72
  tablet preparations 92
  see also beta$_2$-agonists
salmeterol 167–8
sarcoidosis 11, 46
scleroderma 46
screening 102
seasonal asthma 130
secondary asthma 10, 11

sodium cromoglycate 84–5
in adolescence 124
in adult life 130
delivery 96
in drug combinations 89
eye drops 134
in infancy 118–19
spacer devices 94–5
in infancy 118
Spinhaler 96
spirograms 67, 68
spirometry 60–63
equipment 70
and flow-volume measurements 67
method 64
sources of error 65
sputum, asthmatic 21
colour 38
steroid trial 72
stretch receptors 4
submucosal glands 2
innervation 4
sympathetic receptors 76
symptoms 37–8
patterns 103
syrup-based preparations 92, 118
systemic sclerosis 46

tablet preparations 92
teamwork 141–2
terbutaline 77
delivery 96, 99
see also beta$_2$-agonists
theophylline 86–7
administration 87–8
in adolescence 126
in adult life 131
clearance 87
dosage 87–8
in drug combinations 89
in infancy 120
reformulation 75
side effects 88
tablet preparations 92
therapeutic relationship 161
therapeutic tests 71–2, 112
therapy
in adolescence and later childhood 123–8
in adult life 129–33
as crisis intervention 139
in infancy and early childhood 115–20
principles of 107, 110–15
rational approach to 21, 23, 107
tailoring 162–3
trial of 71–2, 110
see also drugs, anti-asthma
tidal volume 64
tobacco smoking
and irreversible airflow limitation 44–5
as trigger factor 33–4
trachea 2
trade names 90
treatment cards 144, 147–9
Tri-flo 96
trigger factors 27–35
Turbohaler 96

underachievement 26
underdiagnosis 24, 102–3
upper respiratory tract
anatomy and physiology 1–2
infections as trigger factors 27, 28–9
urticaria 11, 13, 31

Ventide 89
ventilation 1
control of 6–7
virus infection as trigger factor 28–9
vital capacity 64
Vitalograph 70
Vitalograph Compact 70
Volmax 131
Volumatic 95

weather, role in release of allergens 30
weight gain 129
wheezing 14, 37
in infancy 38, 115
working model 16
Wright peak flow meter 55